MEDCOMIC®
COMPANION
COLORING BOOK

By Jorge Muniz, PA-C

Medcomic: Companion Coloring Book

Copyright © 2015-2018 Medcomic, LLC.

SBN: 978-0-9966513-0-1

Published by Medcomic, LLC.

Director, designer, manager, editor, illustrator, author: Jorge Muniz

CONTENTS

CARDIOVASCULAR

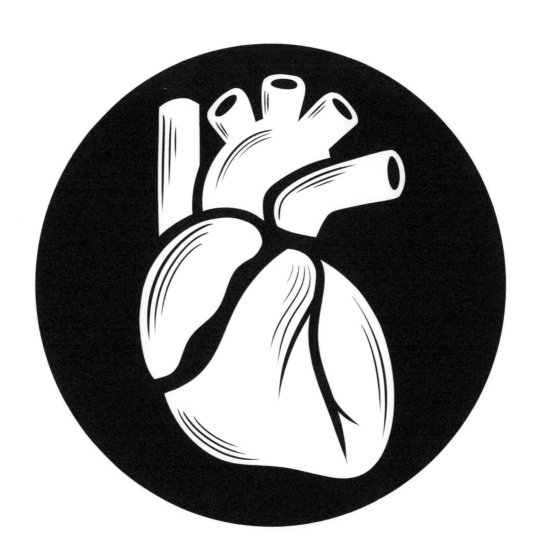

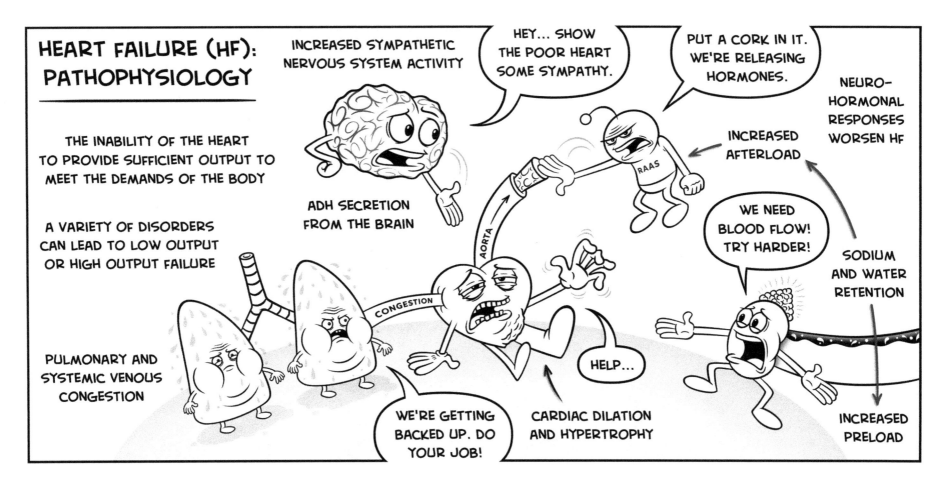

NEW YORK HEART ASSOCIATION (NYHA) HEART FAILURE CLASSIFICATION

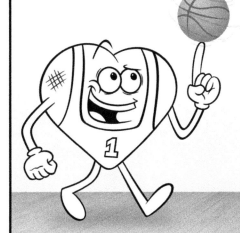

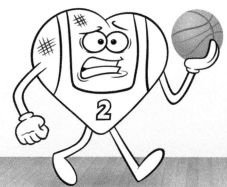

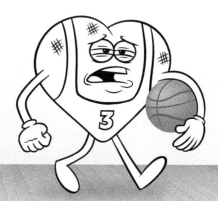

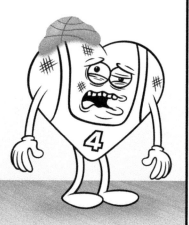

CLASS I	CLASS II	CLASS III	CLASS IV
NO LIMITATION OF PHYSICAL ACTIVITY; ORDINARY PHYSICAL ACTIVITY DOES NOT CAUSE SYMPTOMS	SLIGHT LIMITATION OF PHYSICAL ACTIVITY; COMFORTABLE AT REST; ORDINARY PHYSICAL ACTIVITY CAUSES SYMPTOMS	MARKED LIMITATION OF PHYSICAL ACTIVITY; COMFORTABLE AT REST, BUT LESS THAN ORDINARY ACTIVITY CAUSES SYMPTOMS	SEVERE LIMITATION AND DISCOMFORT WITH ANY PHYSICAL ACTIVITY; SYMPTOMS PRESENT EVEN AT REST

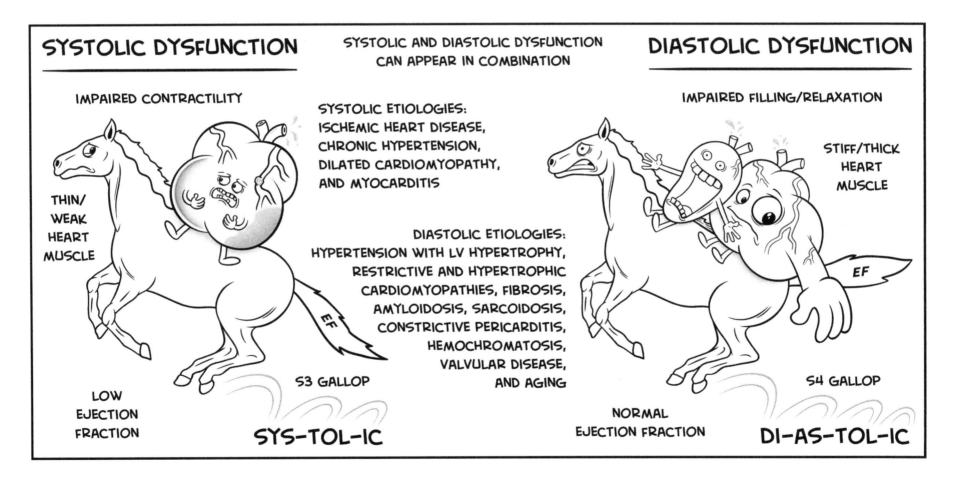

SYSTOLIC DYSFUNCTION

SYSTOLIC AND DIASTOLIC DYSFUNCTION CAN APPEAR IN COMBINATION

DIASTOLIC DYSFUNCTION

IMPAIRED CONTRACTILITY

IMPAIRED FILLING/RELAXATION

SYSTOLIC ETIOLOGIES: ISCHEMIC HEART DISEASE, CHRONIC HYPERTENSION, DILATED CARDIOMYOPATHY, AND MYOCARDITIS

THIN/ WEAK HEART MUSCLE

STIFF/THICK HEART MUSCLE

DIASTOLIC ETIOLOGIES: HYPERTENSION WITH LV HYPERTROPHY, RESTRICTIVE AND HYPERTROPHIC CARDIOMYOPATHIES, FIBROSIS, AMYLOIDOSIS, SARCOIDOSIS, CONSTRICTIVE PERICARDITIS, HEMOCHROMATOSIS, VALVULAR DISEASE, AND AGING

EF

EF

S3 GALLOP

S4 GALLOP

LOW EJECTION FRACTION

SYS-TOL-IC

NORMAL EJECTION FRACTION

DI-AS-TOL-IC

CARDIOMYOPATHY

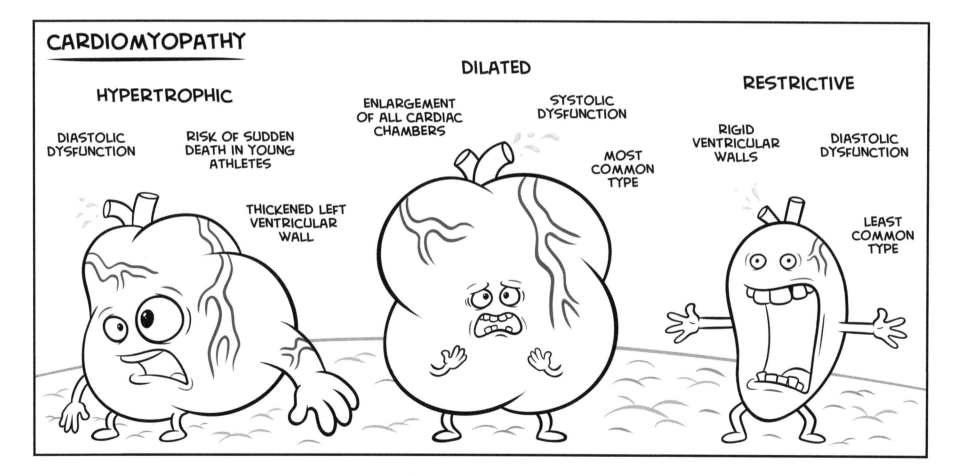

HYPERTROPHIC

DIASTOLIC DYSFUNCTION

RISK OF SUDDEN DEATH IN YOUNG ATHLETES

THICKENED LEFT VENTRICULAR WALL

DILATED

ENLARGEMENT OF ALL CARDIAC CHAMBERS

SYSTOLIC DYSFUNCTION

MOST COMMON TYPE

RESTRICTIVE

RIGID VENTRICULAR WALLS

DIASTOLIC DYSFUNCTION

LEAST COMMON TYPE

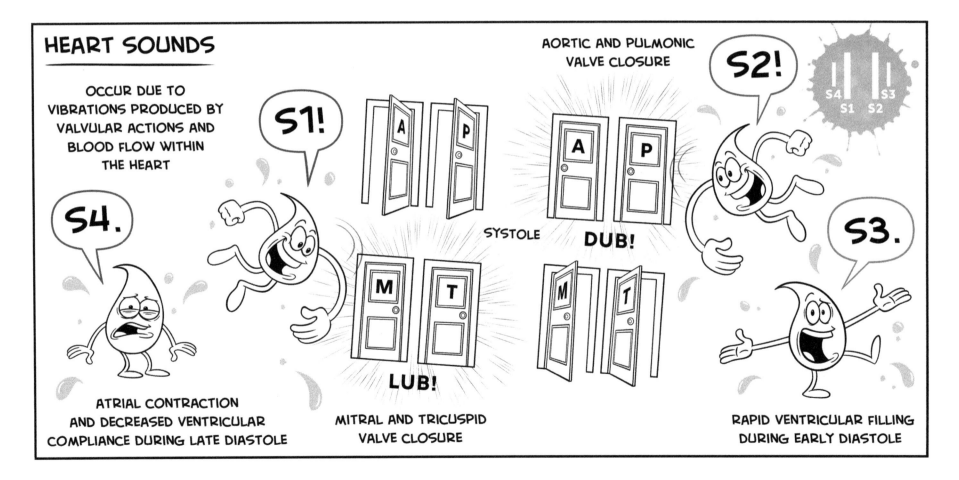

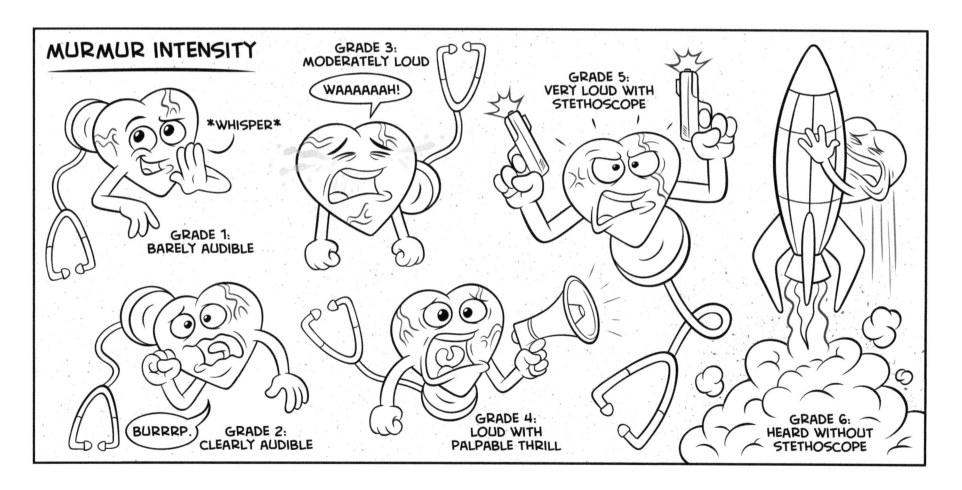

AORTIC STENOSIS

NARROWING AND CALCIFICATION
OF THE AORTIC VALVE RESULTS IN LEFT
VENTRICULAR OUTFLOW OBSTRUCTION

TESTS:
- ECG: LVH, ST-T WAVE CHANGES
- ECHO: CHECK STRUCTURES
  AND PRESSURE GRADIENT
- CARDIAC CATH: ASSESS VALVE
  AREA AND CORONARY
  ARTERIES

THREE MAIN CAUSES:
- CALCIFIC DISEASE OF A TRILEAFLET VALVE
- CALCIFICATION OF A BICUSPID VALVE
- RHEUMATIC VALVE DISEASE

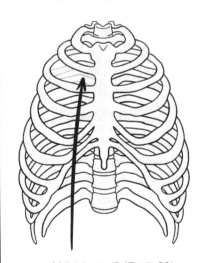

SYSTOLIC EJECTION
MURMUR AT RIGHT SECOND
INTERCOSTAL SPACE

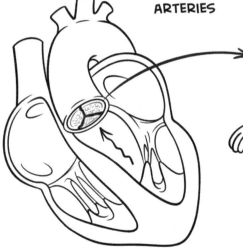

POSSIBLE HEART FAILURE,
ANGINA, AND SYNCOPE

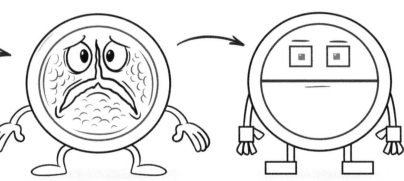

INTERVENTION:
- SURGICAL AORTIC VALVE REPLACEMENT,
- TRANSCATHETER AORTIC VALVE REPLACEMENT
- BALLOON VALVULOPLASTY IN YOUNG PATIENTS
  OR POOR SURGICAL CANDIDATES

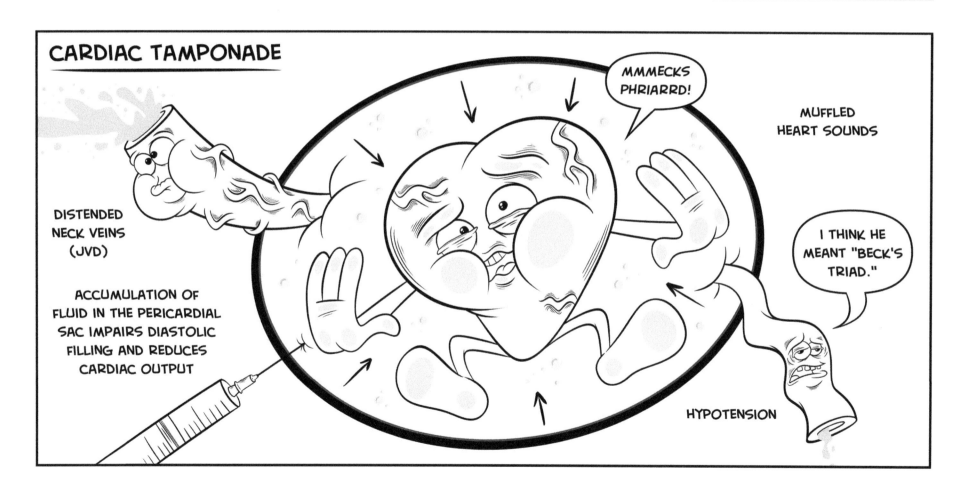

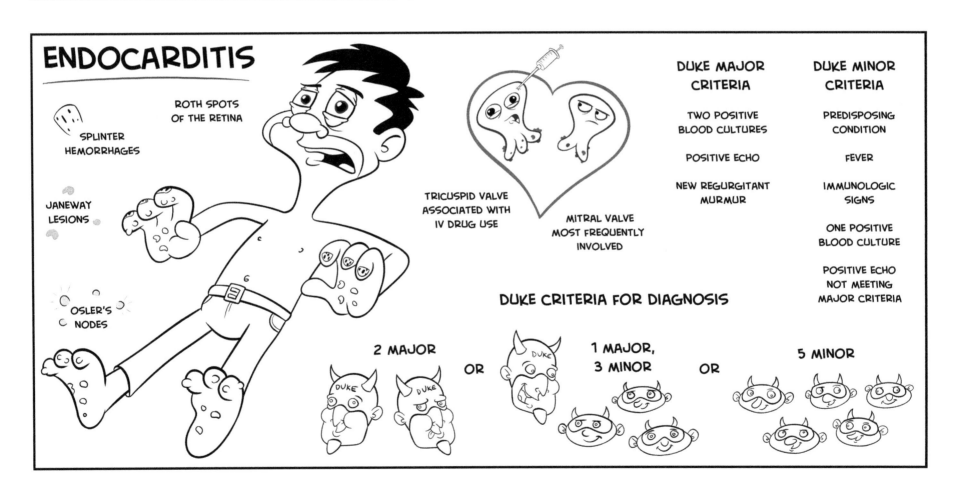

ENDOCARDITIS

SPLINTER HEMORRHAGES

ROTH SPOTS OF THE RETINA

JANEWAY LESIONS

OSLER'S NODES

TRICUSPID VALVE ASSOCIATED WITH IV DRUG USE

MITRAL VALVE MOST FREQUENTLY INVOLVED

DUKE MAJOR CRITERIA

TWO POSITIVE BLOOD CULTURES

POSITIVE ECHO

NEW REGURGITANT MURMUR

DUKE MINOR CRITERIA

PREDISPOSING CONDITION

FEVER

IMMUNOLOGIC SIGNS

ONE POSITIVE BLOOD CULTURE

POSITIVE ECHO NOT MEETING MAJOR CRITERIA

DUKE CRITERIA FOR DIAGNOSIS

2 MAJOR

OR

1 MAJOR, 3 MINOR

OR

5 MINOR

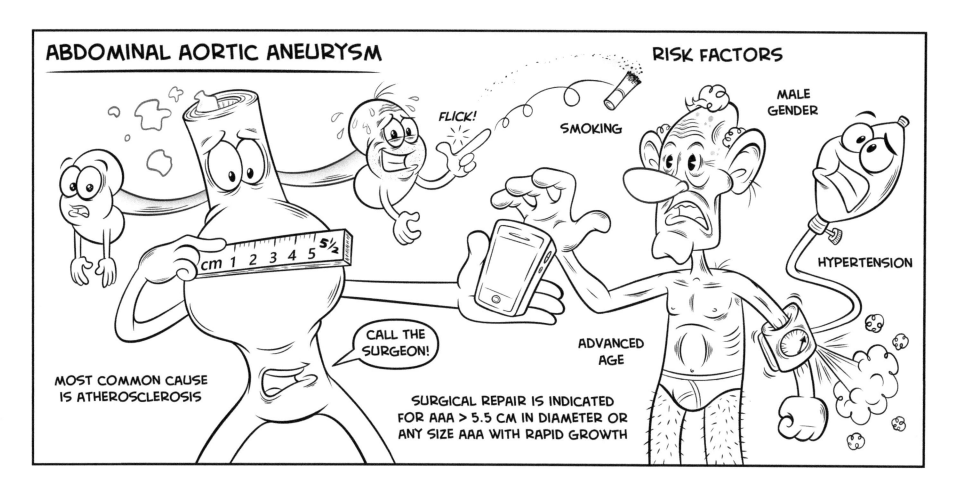

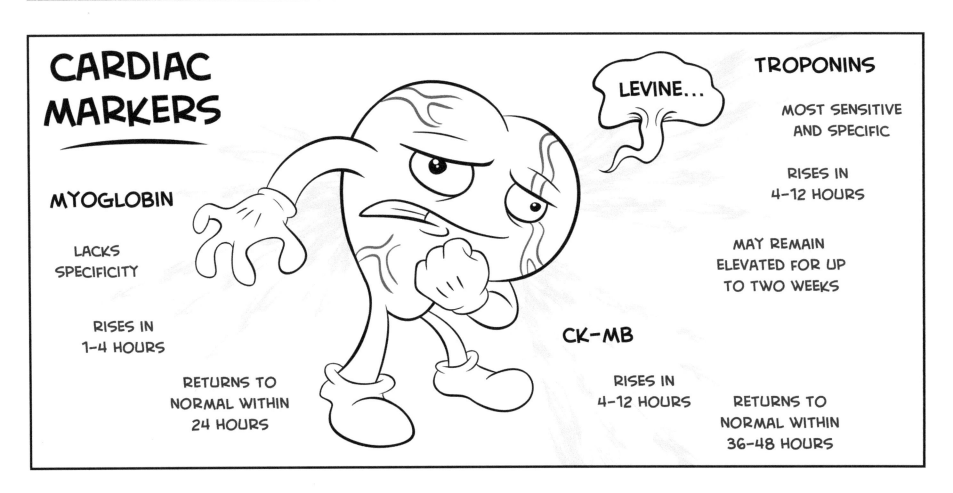

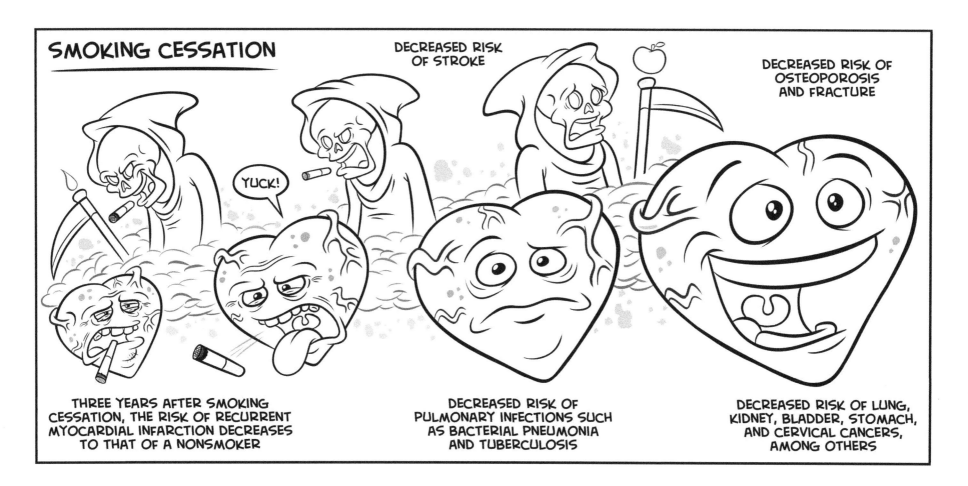

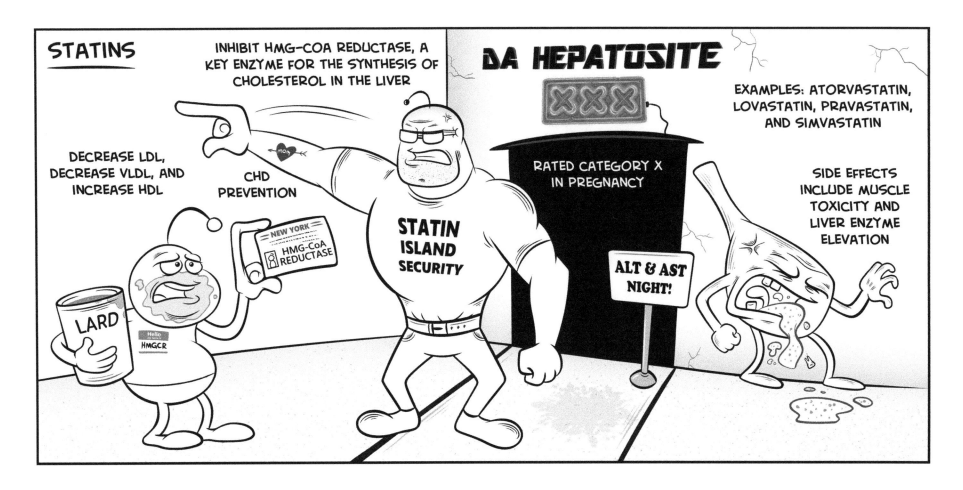

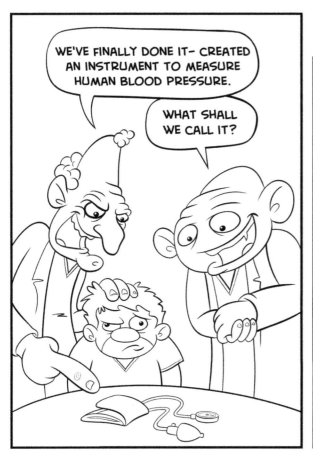
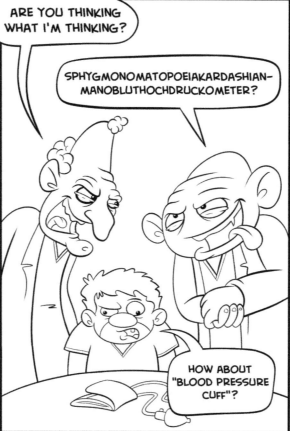
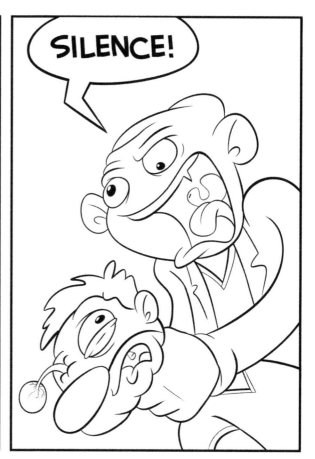

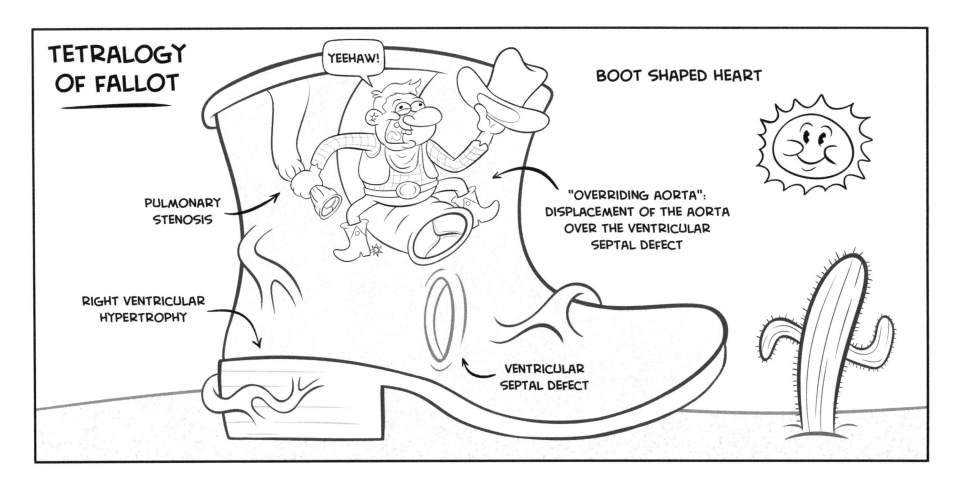

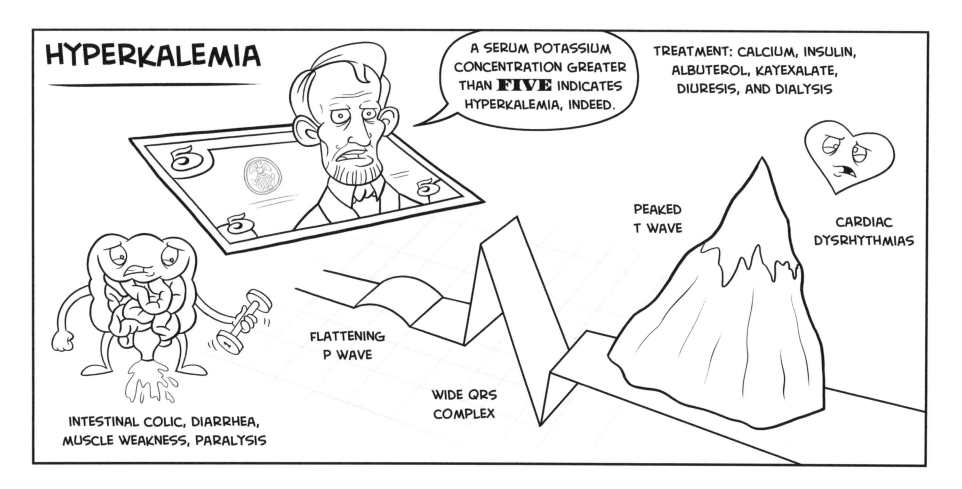

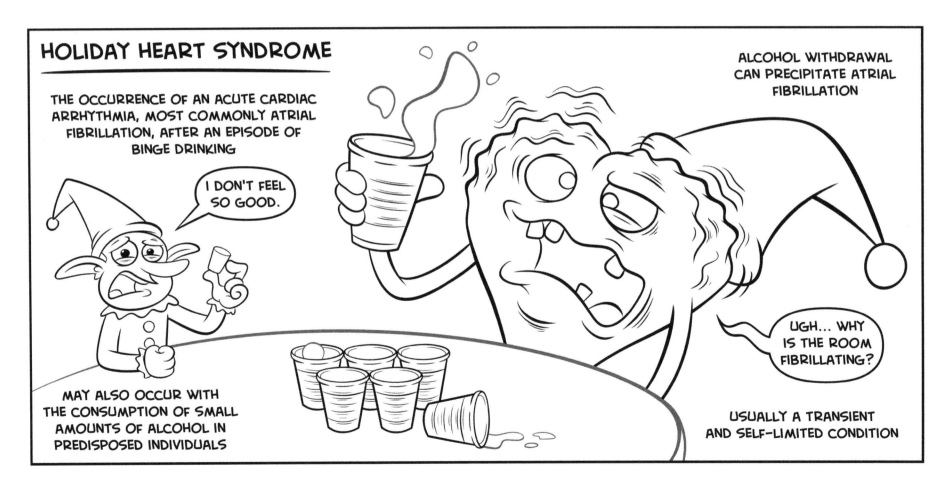

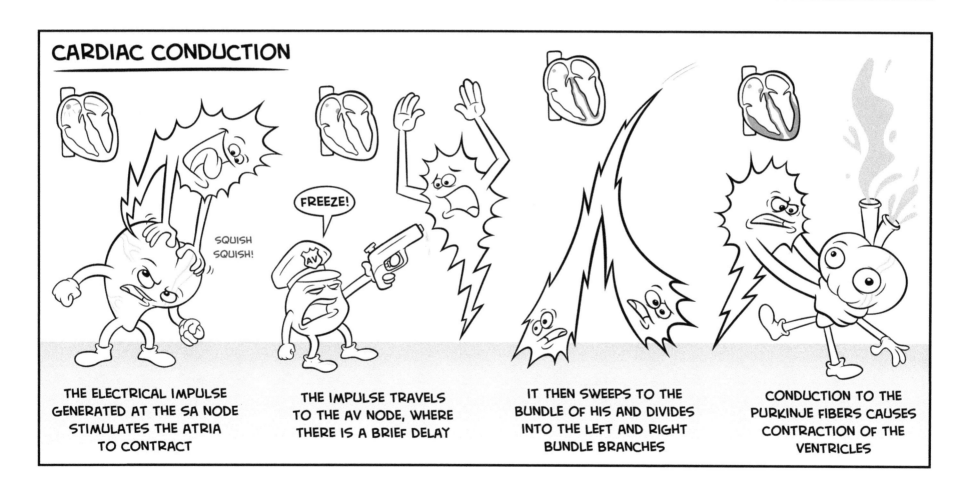

CARDIAC CONDUCTION

THE ELECTRICAL IMPULSE GENERATED AT THE SA NODE STIMULATES THE ATRIA TO CONTRACT

THE IMPULSE TRAVELS TO THE AV NODE, WHERE THERE IS A BRIEF DELAY

IT THEN SWEEPS TO THE BUNDLE OF HIS AND DIVIDES INTO THE LEFT AND RIGHT BUNDLE BRANCHES

CONDUCTION TO THE PURKINJE FIBERS CAUSES CONTRACTION OF THE VENTRICLES

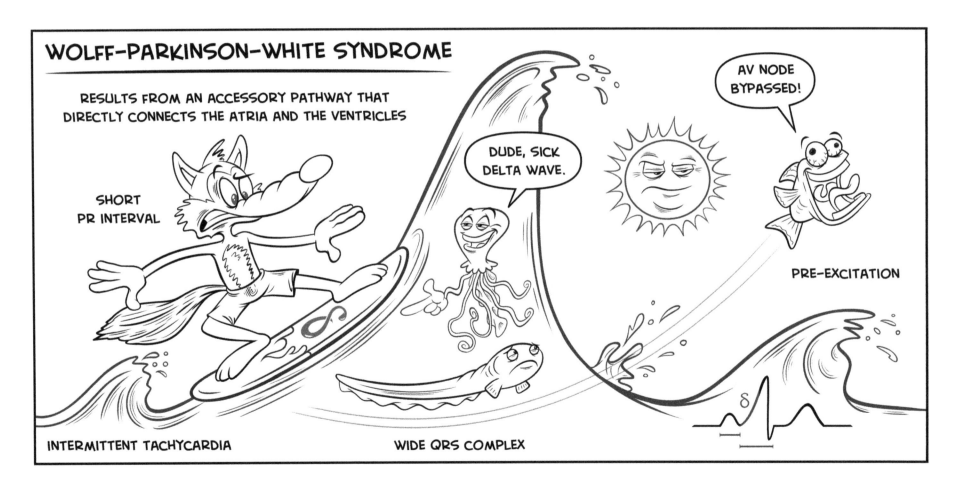

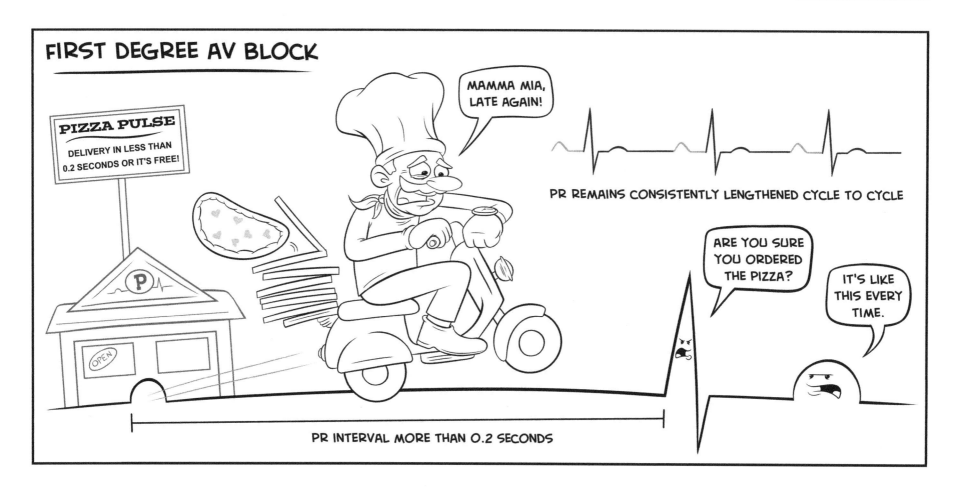

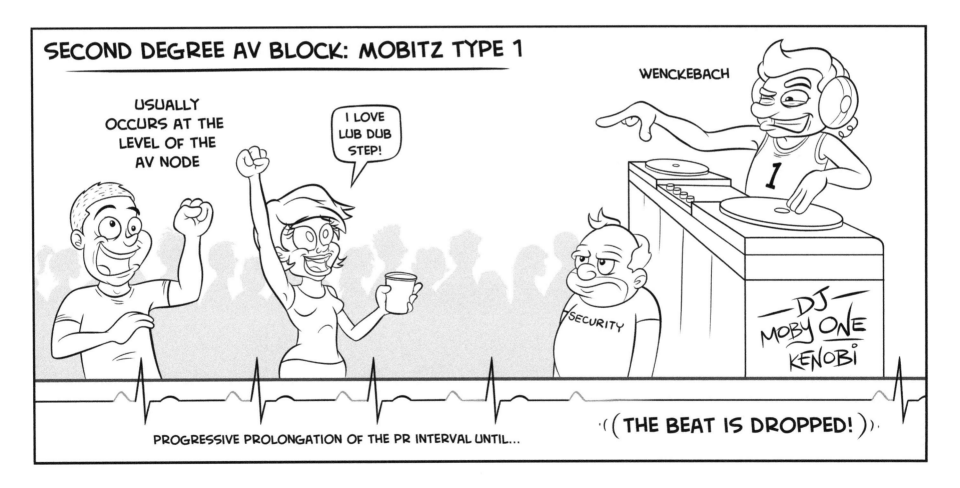

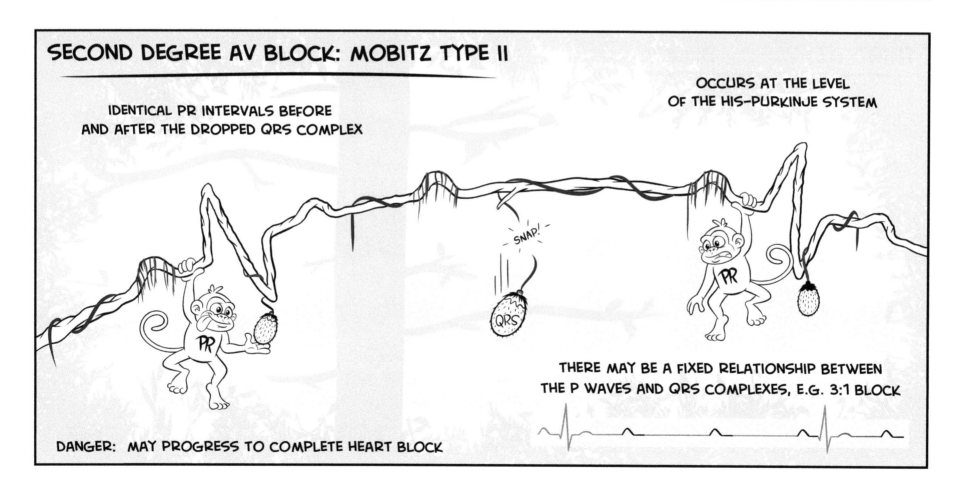

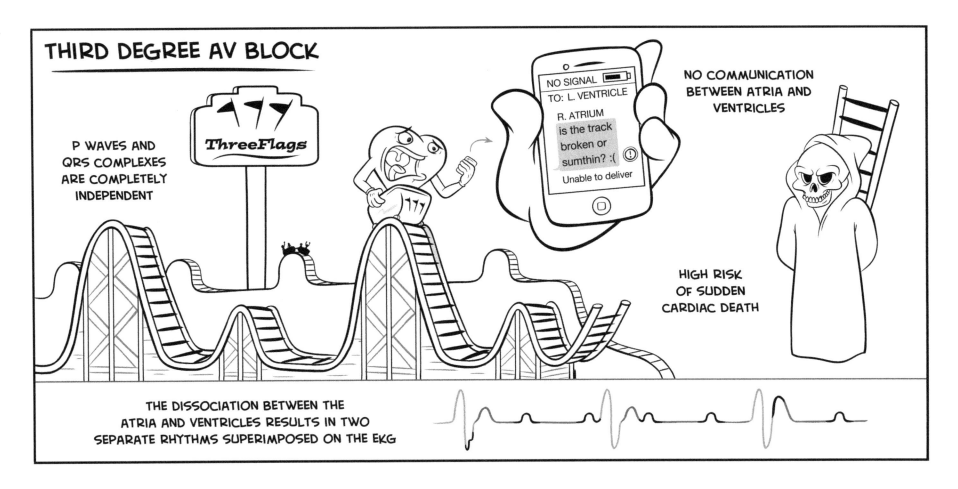

PULMONOLOGY

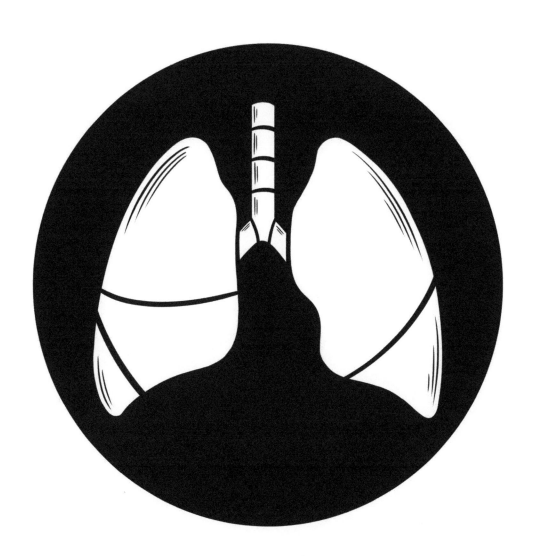

PULMONARY HYPERTENSION

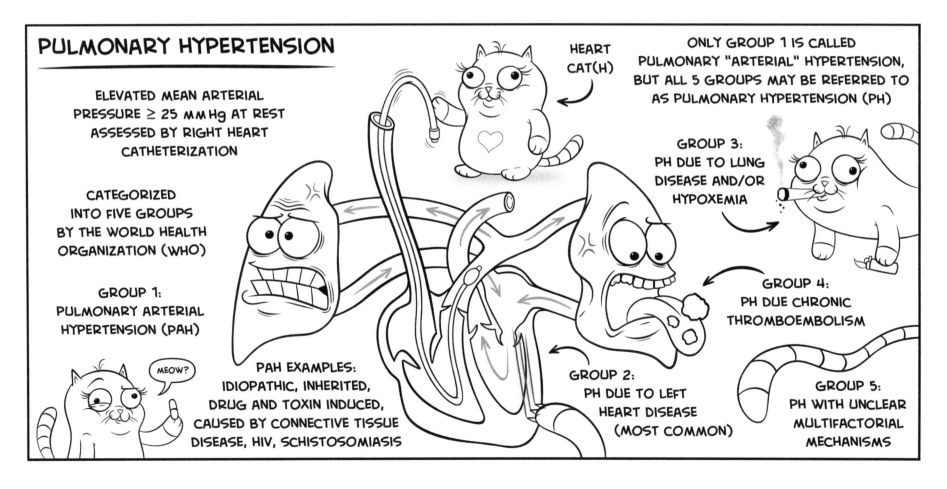

ELEVATED MEAN ARTERIAL PRESSURE ≥ 25 mmHg AT REST ASSESSED BY RIGHT HEART CATHETERIZATION

CATEGORIZED INTO FIVE GROUPS BY THE WORLD HEALTH ORGANIZATION (WHO)

GROUP 1: PULMONARY ARTERIAL HYPERTENSION (PAH)

MEOW?

PAH EXAMPLES: IDIOPATHIC, INHERITED, DRUG AND TOXIN INDUCED, CAUSED BY CONNECTIVE TISSUE DISEASE, HIV, SCHISTOSOMIASIS

HEART CAT(H)

ONLY GROUP 1 IS CALLED PULMONARY "ARTERIAL" HYPERTENSION, BUT ALL 5 GROUPS MAY BE REFERRED TO AS PULMONARY HYPERTENSION (PH)

GROUP 3: PH DUE TO LUNG DISEASE AND/OR HYPOXEMIA

GROUP 4: PH DUE CHRONIC THROMBOEMBOLISM

GROUP 2: PH DUE TO LEFT HEART DISEASE (MOST COMMON)

GROUP 5: PH WITH UNCLEAR MULTIFACTORIAL MECHANISMS

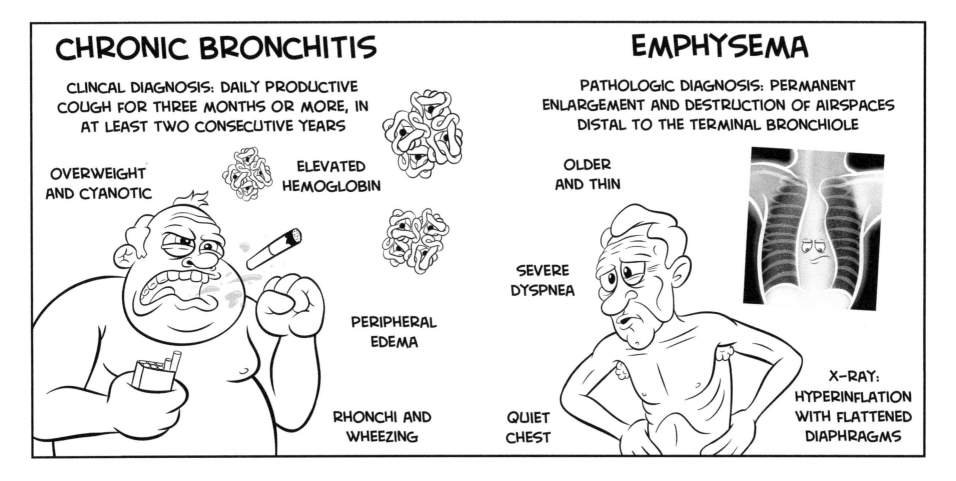

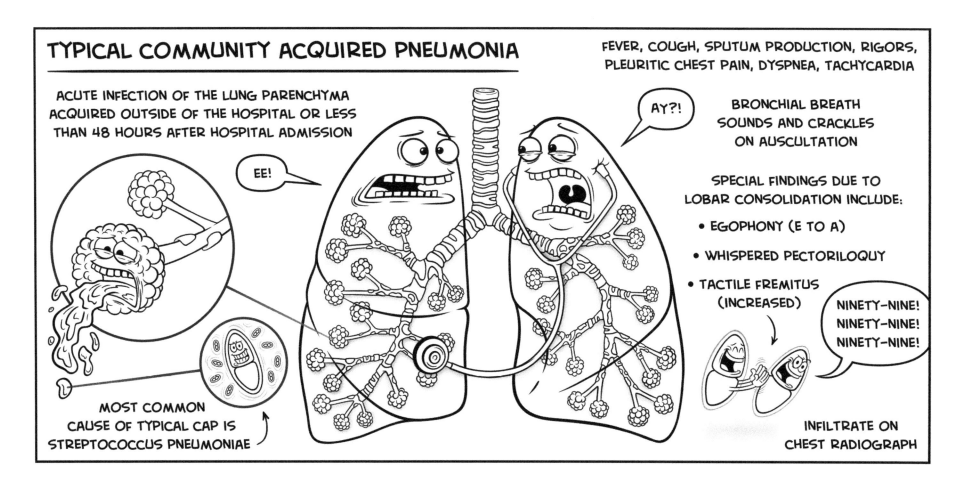

CLASSIFICATION OF ASTHMA

P E R S I S T E N T

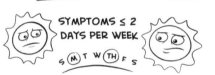

SYMPTOMS ≤ 2 DAYS PER WEEK

S M T W TH F S

RESCUE MEDICATION
< 2 DAYS PER WEEK

NIGHTTIME SYMPTOMS
≤ 2 TIMES PER MONTH

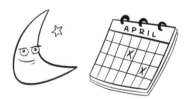

FEV1 > 80% PREDICTED
FEV1/FVC NORMAL

INTERMITTENT

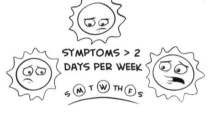

SYMPTOMS > 2 DAYS PER WEEK

S M T W TH F S

RESCUE MEDICATION
> 2 DAYS PER WEEK

NIGHTTIME SYMPTOMS
3–4 TIMES PER MONTH

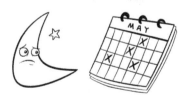

FEV1 > 80% PREDICTED
FEV1/FVC NORMAL

MILD

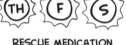

DAILY SYMPTOMS

TH F S

RESCUE MEDICATION
DAILY

NIGHTTIME SYMPTOMS
> 1 TIME PER WEEK

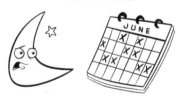

FEV1 > 60% BUT < 80% PREDICTED
FEV1/FVC REDUCED 5%

MODERATE

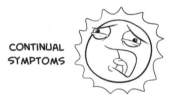

CONTINUAL SYMPTOMS

RESCUE MEDICATION
SEVERAL TIMES PER DAY

NIGHTTIME SYMPTOMS
OFTEN > 7 TIMES PER WEEK

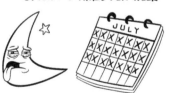

FEV1 < 60% PREDICTED
FEV1/FVC REDUCED > 5%

SEVERE

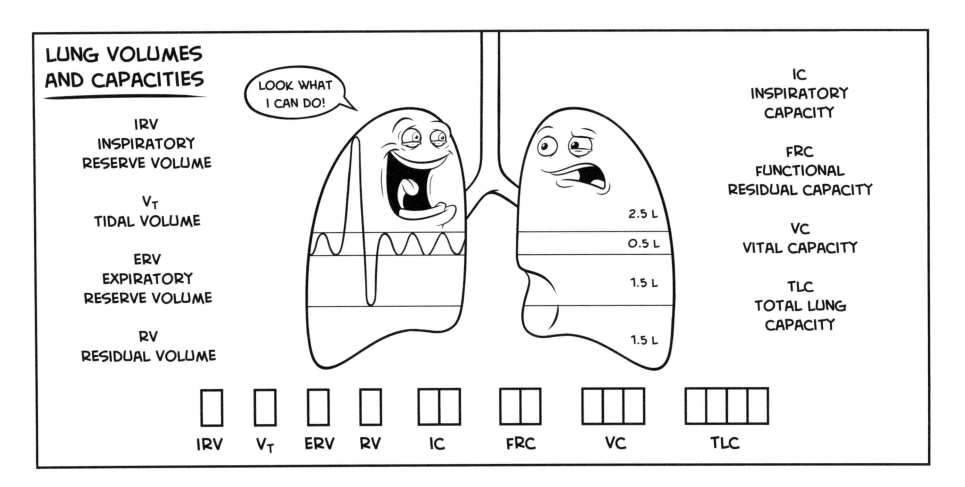

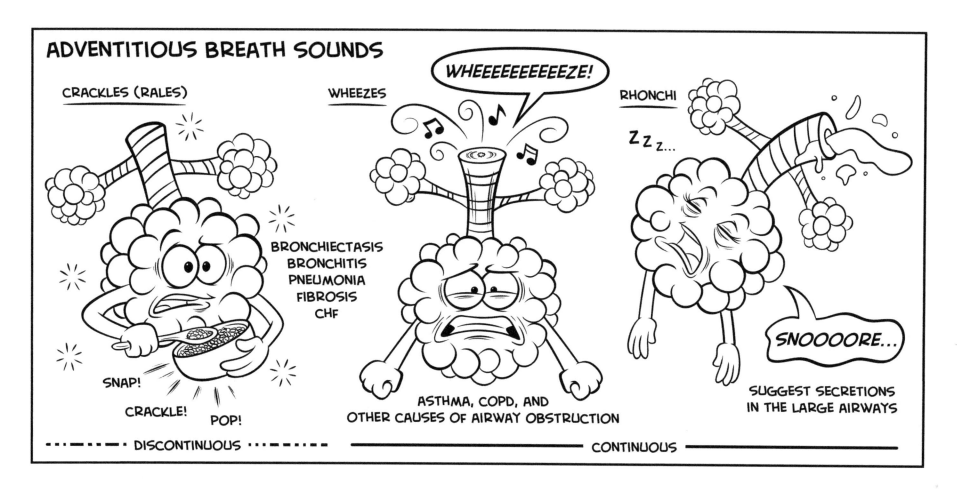

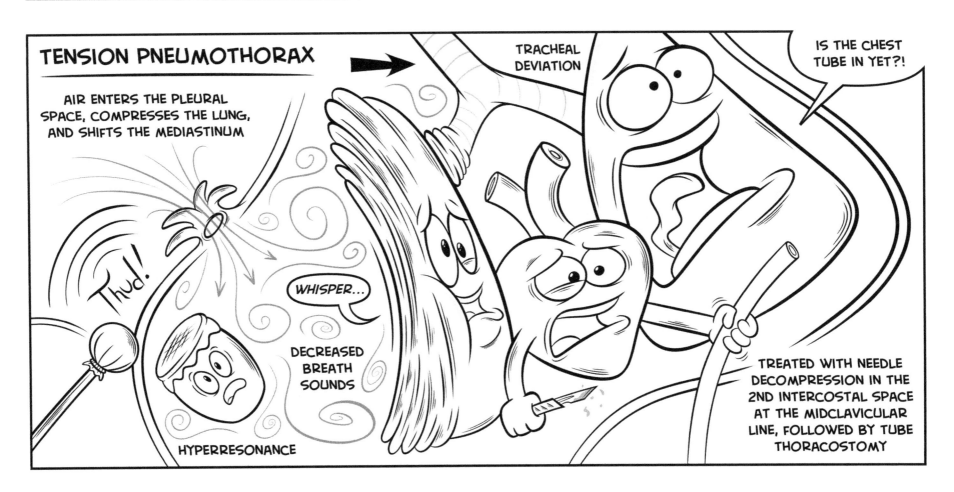

ENDOCRINOLOGY

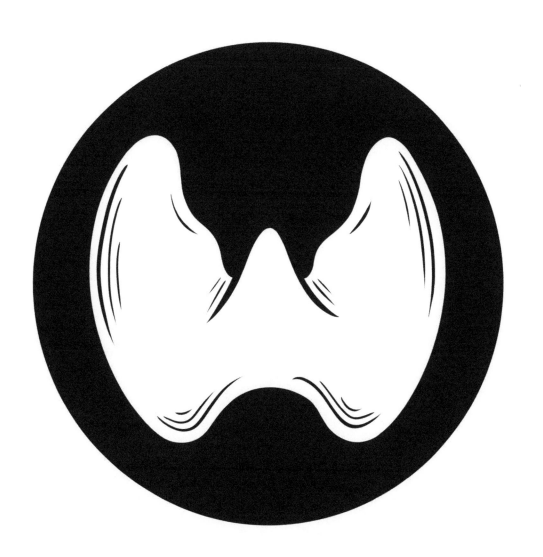

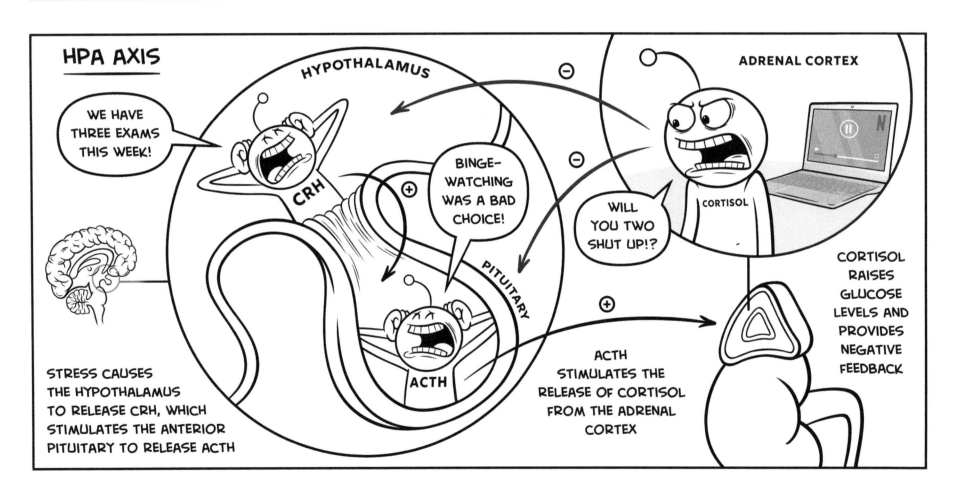

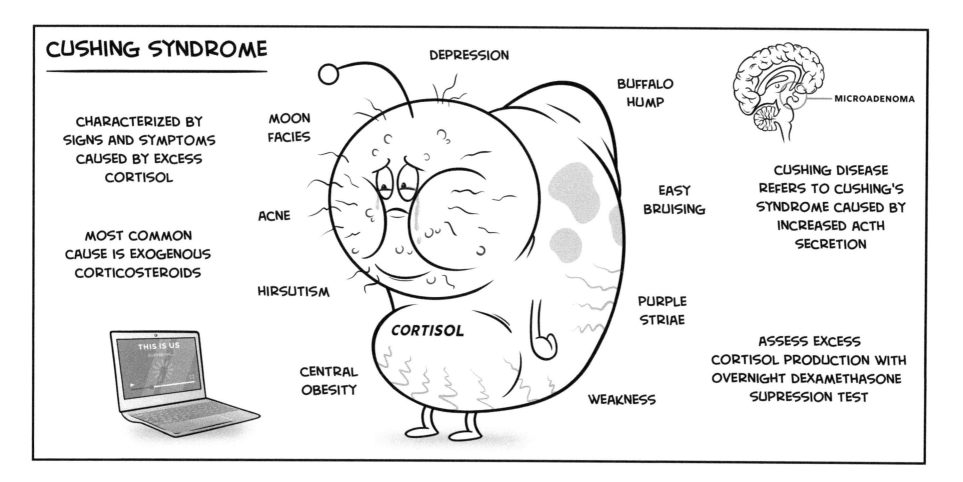

CUSHING SYNDROME

CHARACTERIZED BY SIGNS AND SYMPTOMS CAUSED BY EXCESS CORTISOL

MOST COMMON CAUSE IS EXOGENOUS CORTICOSTEROIDS

DEPRESSION

MOON FACIES

ACNE

HIRSUTISM

CENTRAL OBESITY

CORTISOL

THIS IS US

BUFFALO HUMP

EASY BRUISING

PURPLE STRIAE

WEAKNESS

MICROADENOMA

CUSHING DISEASE REFERS TO CUSHING'S SYNDROME CAUSED BY INCREASED ACTH SECRETION

ASSESS EXCESS CORTISOL PRODUCTION WITH OVERNIGHT DEXAMETHASONE SUPRESSION TEST

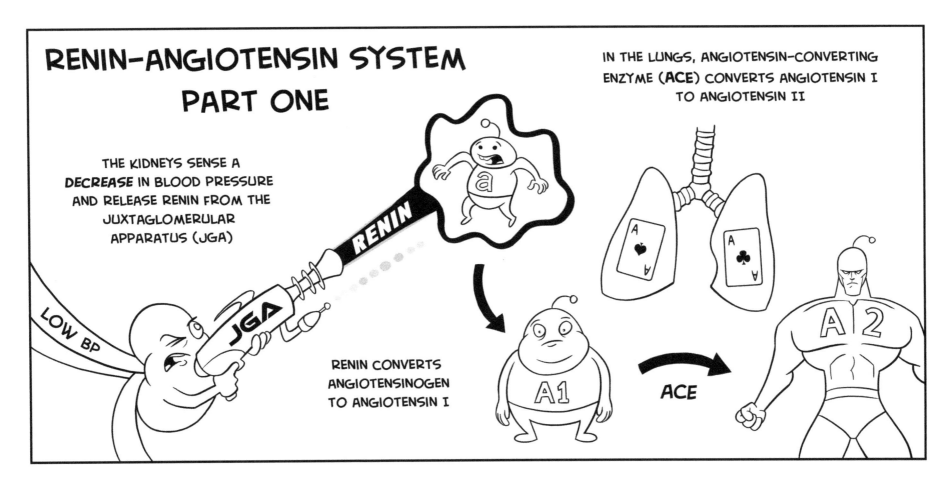

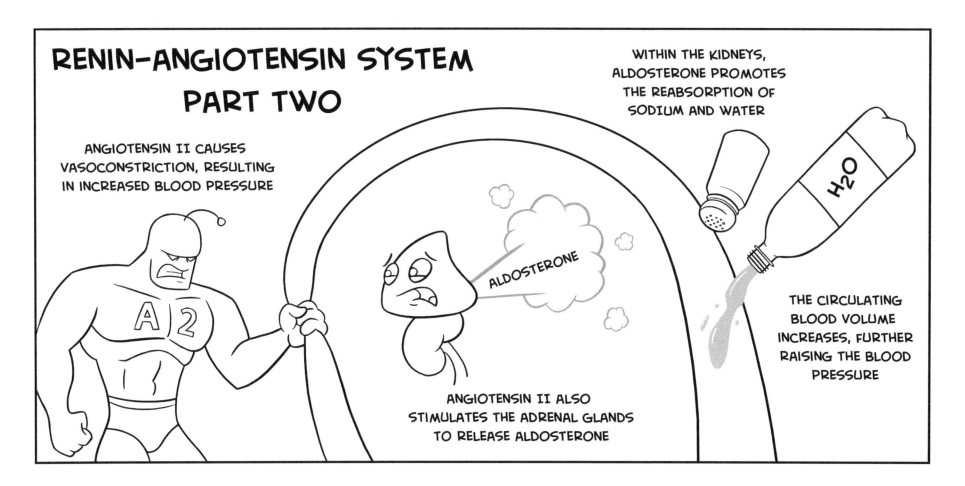

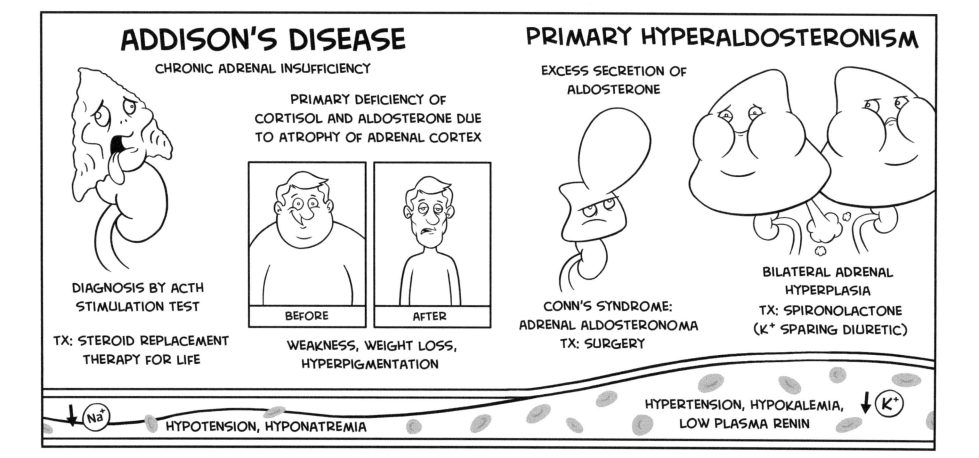

ADDISON'S DISEASE

CHRONIC ADRENAL INSUFFICIENCY

PRIMARY DEFICIENCY OF CORTISOL AND ALDOSTERONE DUE TO ATROPHY OF ADRENAL CORTEX

BEFORE

AFTER

DIAGNOSIS BY ACTH STIMULATION TEST

TX: STEROID REPLACEMENT THERAPY FOR LIFE

WEAKNESS, WEIGHT LOSS, HYPERPIGMENTATION

PRIMARY HYPERALDOSTERONISM

EXCESS SECRETION OF ALDOSTERONE

BILATERAL ADRENAL HYPERPLASIA

TX: SPIRONOLACTONE (K⁺ SPARING DIURETIC)

CONN'S SYNDROME: ADRENAL ALDOSTERONOMA

TX: SURGERY

HYPOTENSION, HYPONATREMIA

HYPERTENSION, HYPOKALEMIA, LOW PLASMA RENIN

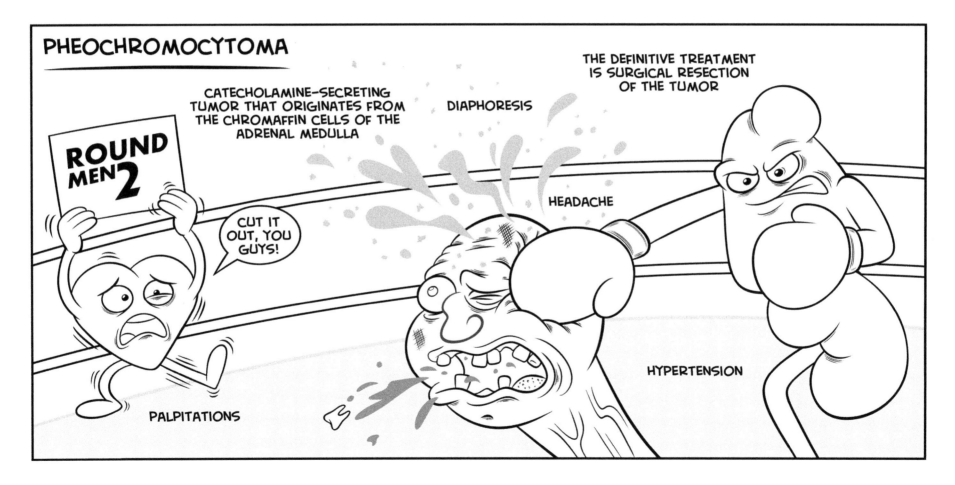

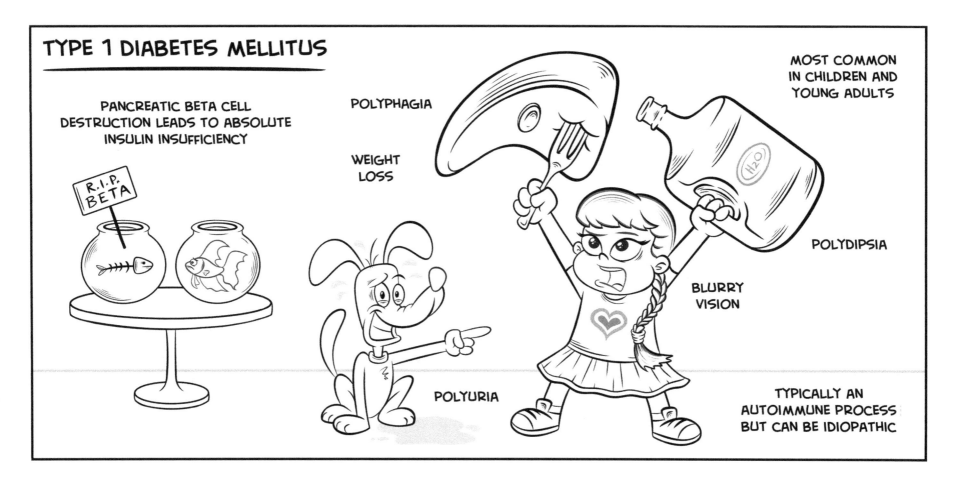

TYPE 1 DIABETES MELLITUS

PANCREATIC BETA CELL DESTRUCTION LEADS TO ABSOLUTE INSULIN INSUFFICIENCY

POLYPHAGIA

WEIGHT LOSS

MOST COMMON IN CHILDREN AND YOUNG ADULTS

R.I.P. BETA

H2O

POLYDIPSIA

BLURRY VISION

POLYURIA

TYPICALLY AN AUTOIMMUNE PROCESS BUT CAN BE IDIOPATHIC

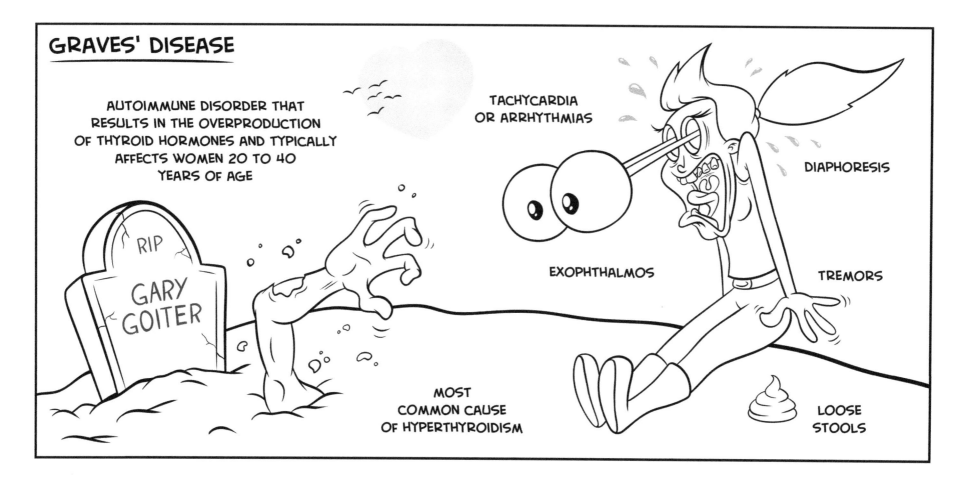

GRAVES' DISEASE

AUTOIMMUNE DISORDER THAT RESULTS IN THE OVERPRODUCTION OF THYROID HORMONES AND TYPICALLY AFFECTS WOMEN 20 TO 40 YEARS OF AGE

RIP GARY GOITER

MOST COMMON CAUSE OF HYPERTHYROIDISM

TACHYCARDIA OR ARRHYTHMIAS

EXOPHTHALMOS

DIAPHORESIS

TREMORS

LOOSE STOOLS

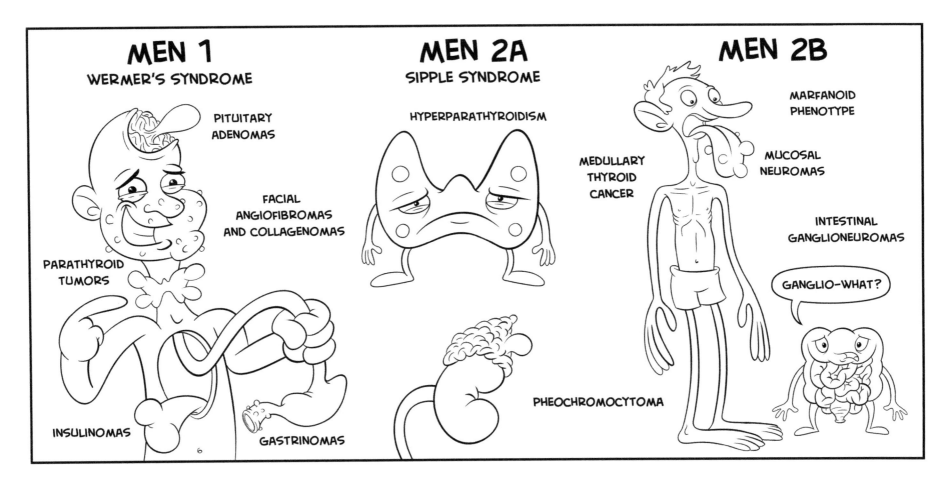

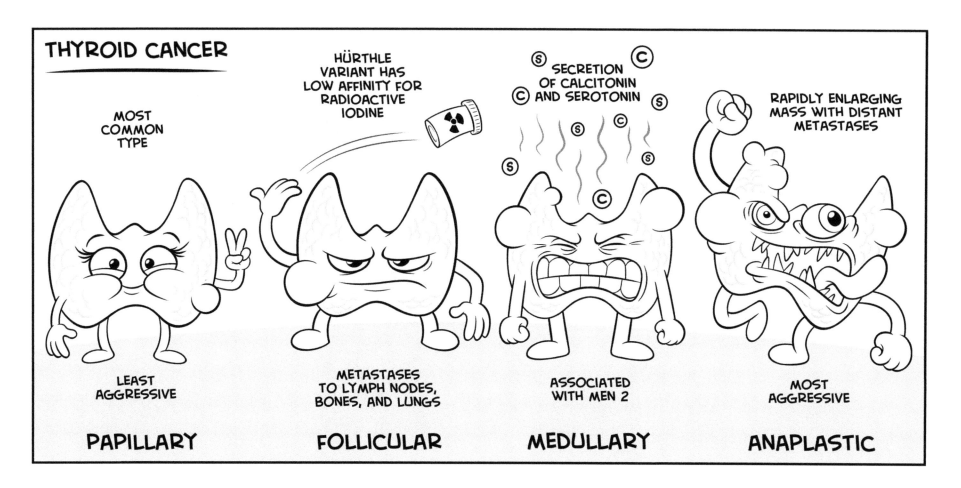

THYROID CANCER

PAPILLARY
MOST COMMON TYPE
LEAST AGGRESSIVE

FOLLICULAR
HÜRTHLE VARIANT HAS LOW AFFINITY FOR RADIOACTIVE IODINE
METASTASES TO LYMPH NODES, BONES, AND LUNGS

MEDULLARY
SECRETION OF CALCITONIN AND SEROTONIN
ASSOCIATED WITH MEN 2

ANAPLASTIC
RAPIDLY ENLARGING MASS WITH DISTANT METASTASES
MOST AGGRESSIVE

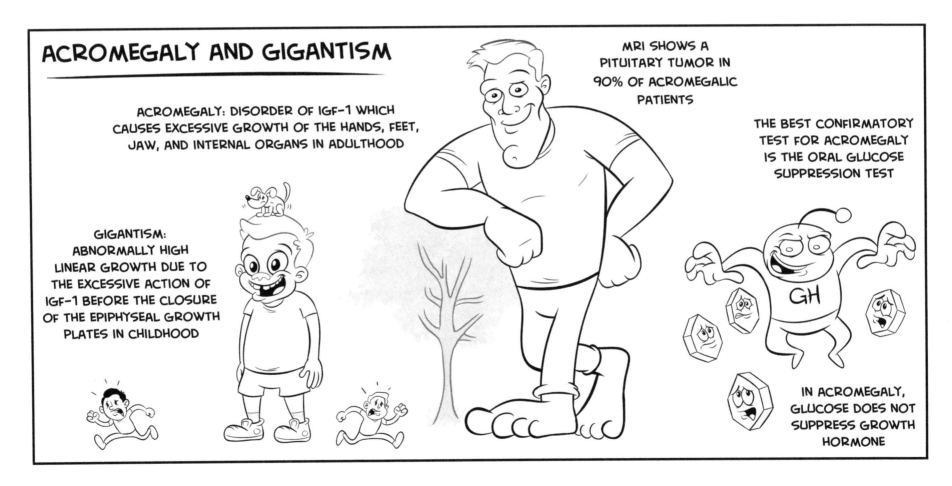

ACROMEGALY AND GIGANTISM

ACROMEGALY: DISORDER OF IGF-1 WHICH CAUSES EXCESSIVE GROWTH OF THE HANDS, FEET, JAW, AND INTERNAL ORGANS IN ADULTHOOD

GIGANTISM: ABNORMALLY HIGH LINEAR GROWTH DUE TO THE EXCESSIVE ACTION OF IGF-1 BEFORE THE CLOSURE OF THE EPIPHYSEAL GROWTH PLATES IN CHILDHOOD

MRI SHOWS A PITUITARY TUMOR IN 90% OF ACROMEGALIC PATIENTS

THE BEST CONFIRMATORY TEST FOR ACROMEGALY IS THE ORAL GLUCOSE SUPPRESSION TEST

GH

IN ACROMEGALY, GLUCOSE DOES NOT SUPPRESS GROWTH HORMONE

SURGERY

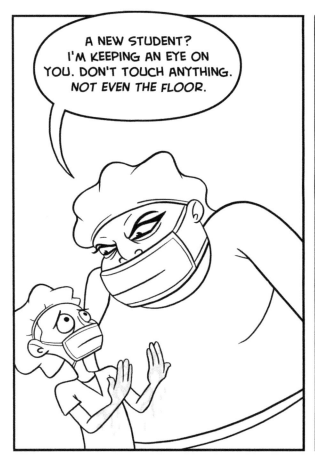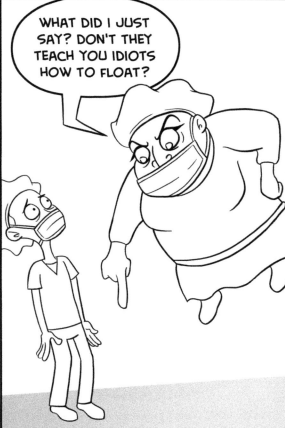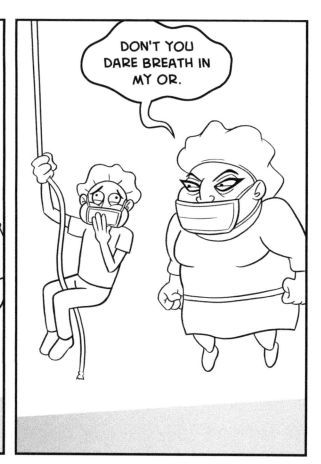

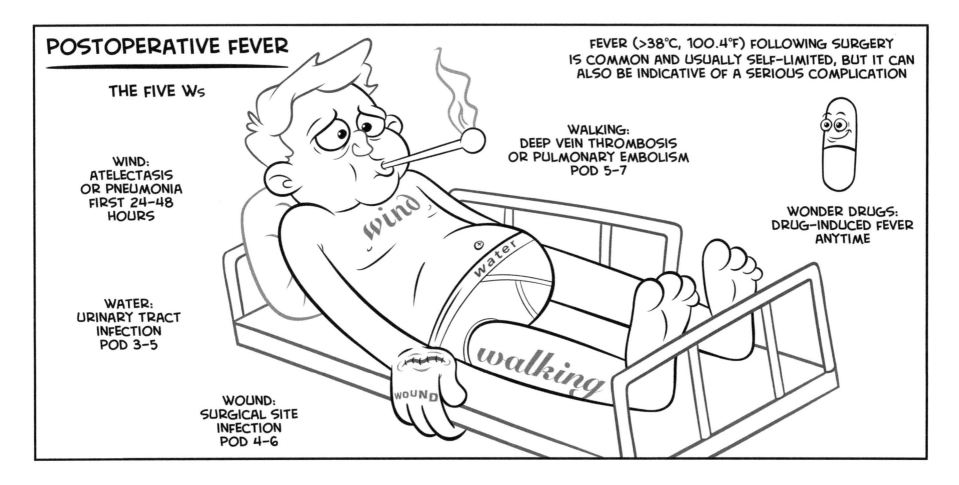

POSTOPERATIVE FEVER

FEVER (>38°C, 100.4°F) FOLLOWING SURGERY IS COMMON AND USUALLY SELF-LIMITED, BUT IT CAN ALSO BE INDICATIVE OF A SERIOUS COMPLICATION

THE FIVE Ws

WIND:
ATELECTASIS
OR PNEUMONIA
FIRST 24-48
HOURS

WATER:
URINARY TRACT
INFECTION
POD 3-5

WOUND:
SURGICAL SITE
INFECTION
POD 4-6

WALKING:
DEEP VEIN THROMBOSIS
OR PULMONARY EMBOLISM
POD 5-7

WONDER DRUGS:
DRUG-INDUCED FEVER
ANYTIME

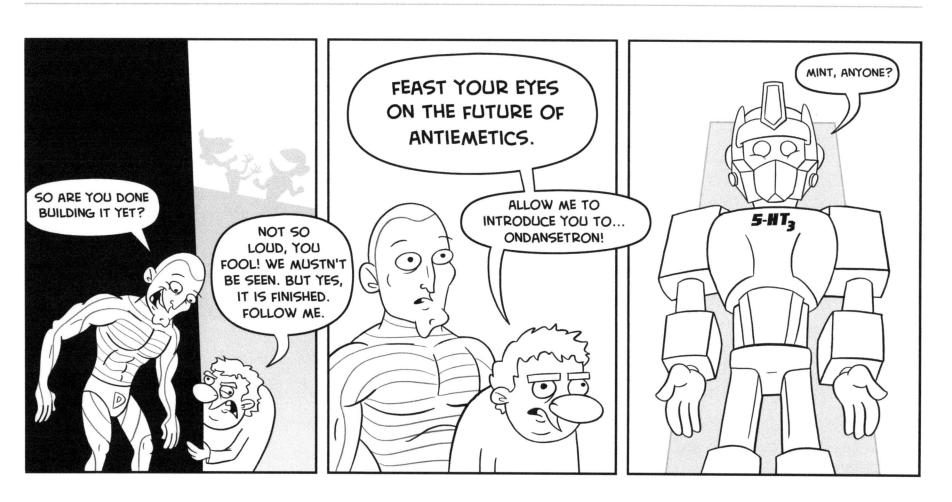

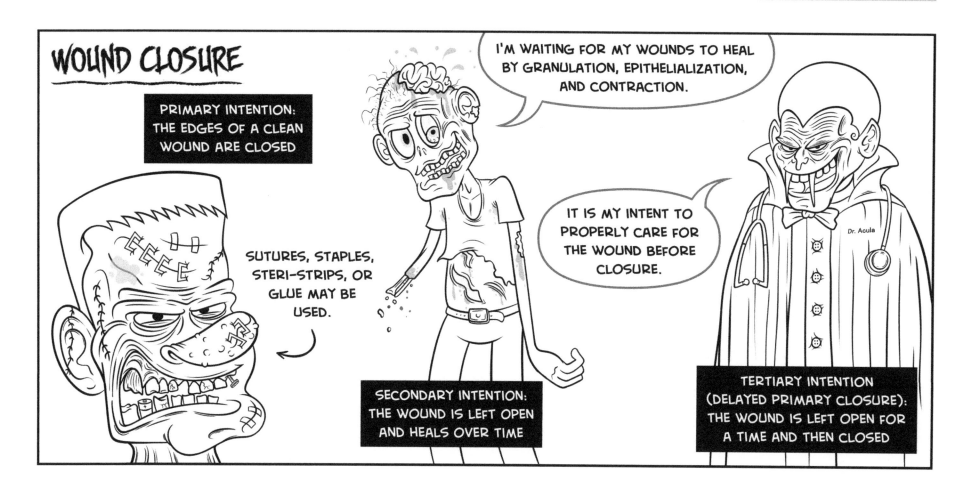

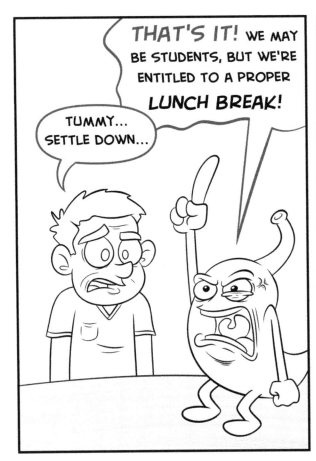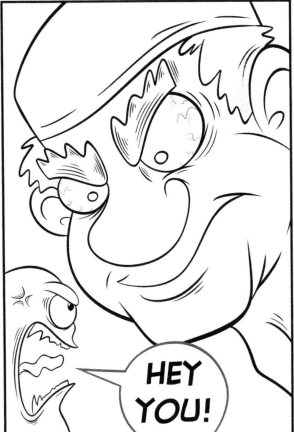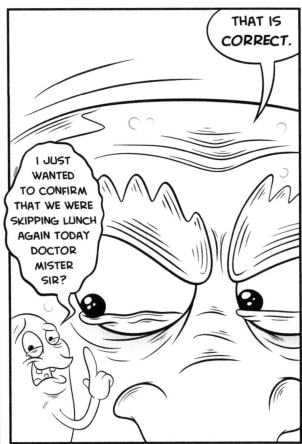

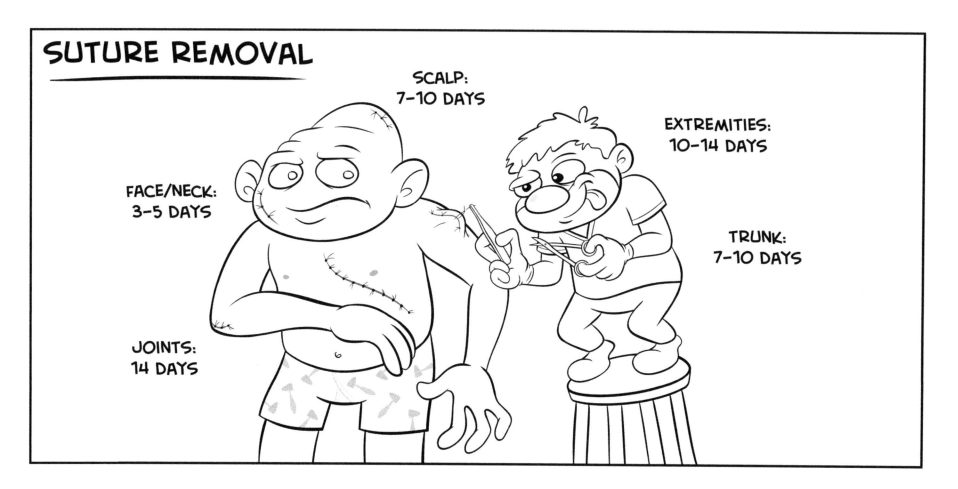

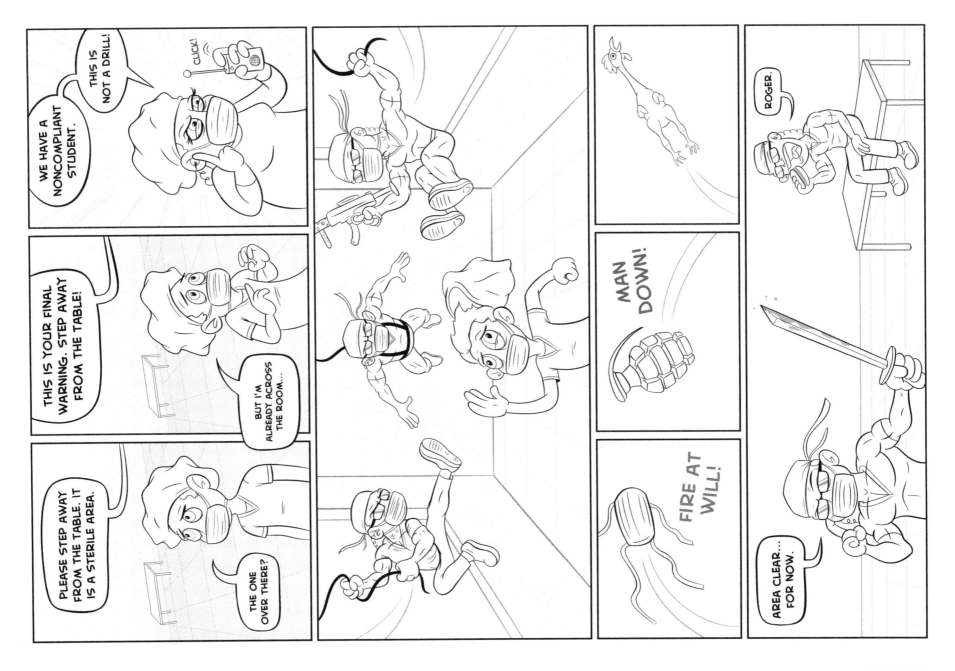

INFECTIOUS DISEASE

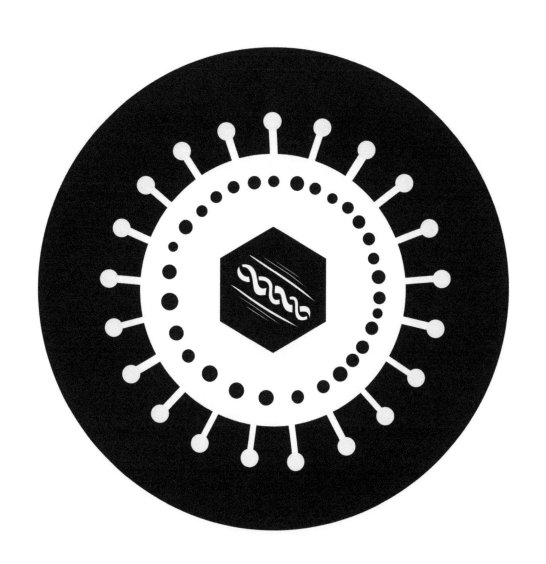

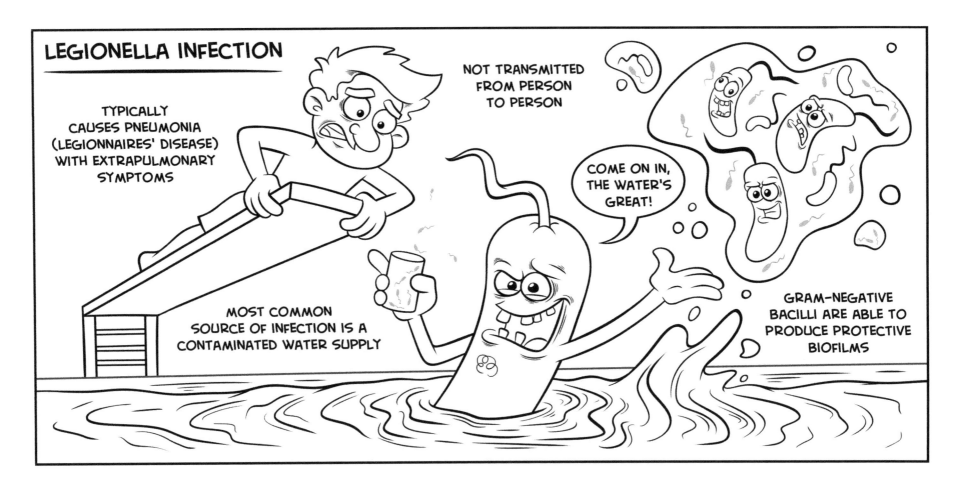

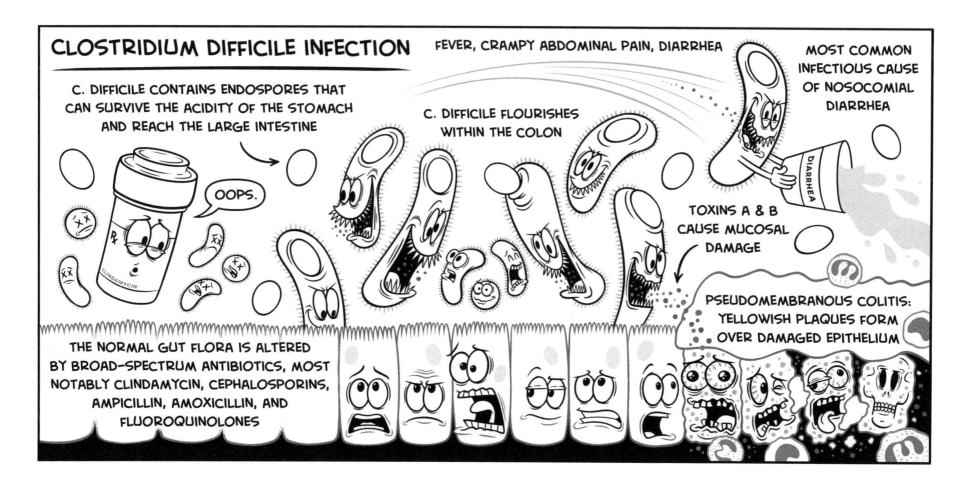

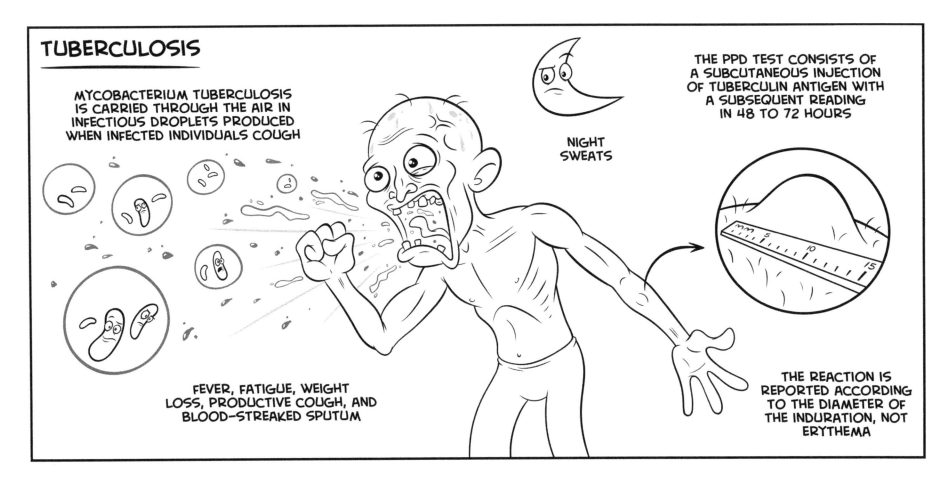

TUBERCULOSIS

MYCOBACTERIUM TUBERCULOSIS IS CARRIED THROUGH THE AIR IN INFECTIOUS DROPLETS PRODUCED WHEN INFECTED INDIVIDUALS COUGH

NIGHT SWEATS

THE PPD TEST CONSISTS OF A SUBCUTANEOUS INJECTION OF TUBERCULIN ANTIGEN WITH A SUBSEQUENT READING IN 48 TO 72 HOURS

FEVER, FATIGUE, WEIGHT LOSS, PRODUCTIVE COUGH, AND BLOOD-STREAKED SPUTUM

THE REACTION IS REPORTED ACCORDING TO THE DIAMETER OF THE INDURATION, NOT ERYTHEMA

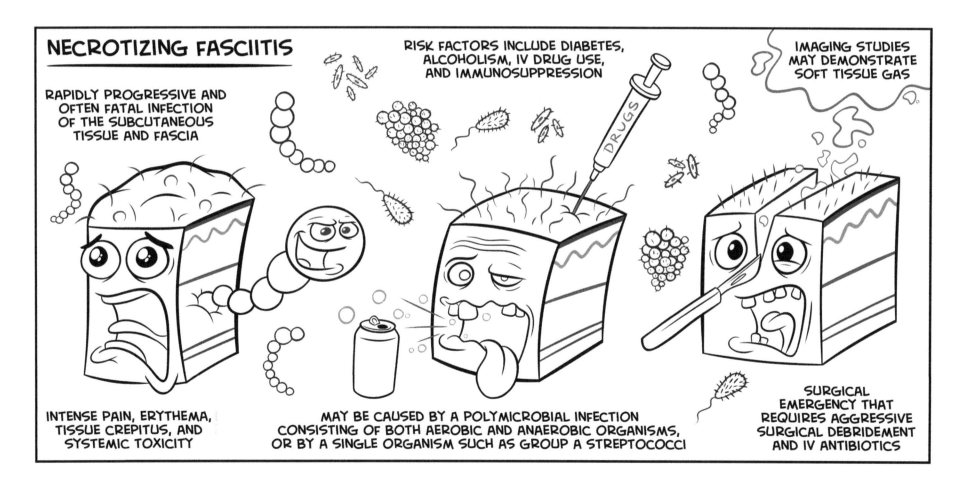

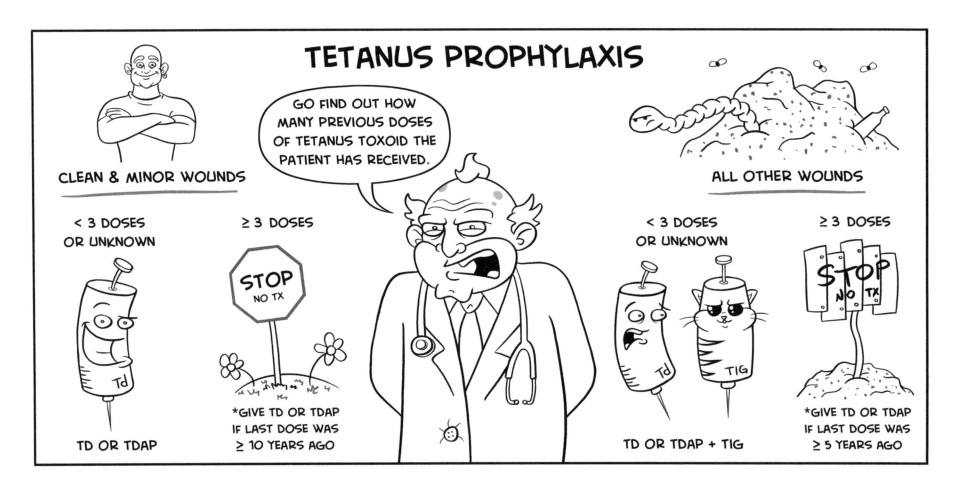

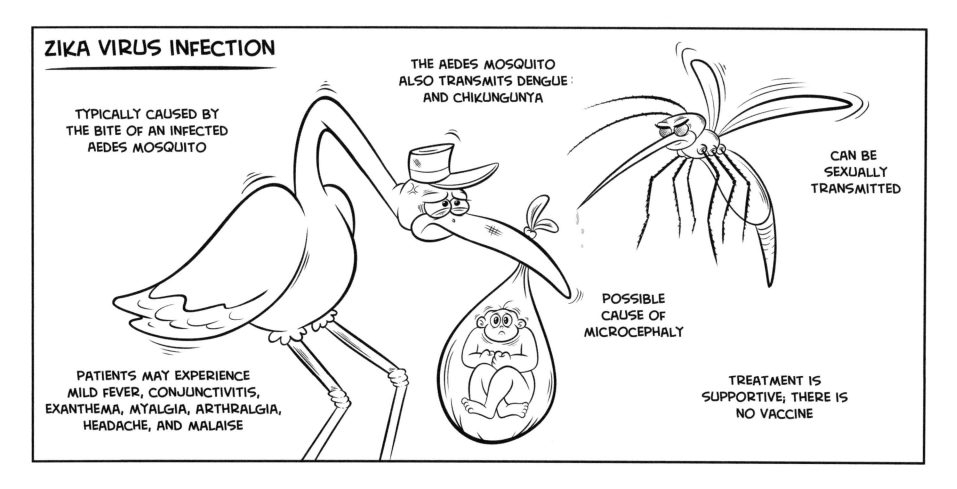

ZIKA VIRUS INFECTION

TYPICALLY CAUSED BY THE BITE OF AN INFECTED AEDES MOSQUITO

THE AEDES MOSQUITO ALSO TRANSMITS DENGUE AND CHIKUNGUNYA

CAN BE SEXUALLY TRANSMITTED

POSSIBLE CAUSE OF MICROCEPHALY

PATIENTS MAY EXPERIENCE MILD FEVER, CONJUNCTIVITIS, EXANTHEMA, MYALGIA, ARTHRALGIA, HEADACHE, AND MALAISE

TREATMENT IS SUPPORTIVE; THERE IS NO VACCINE

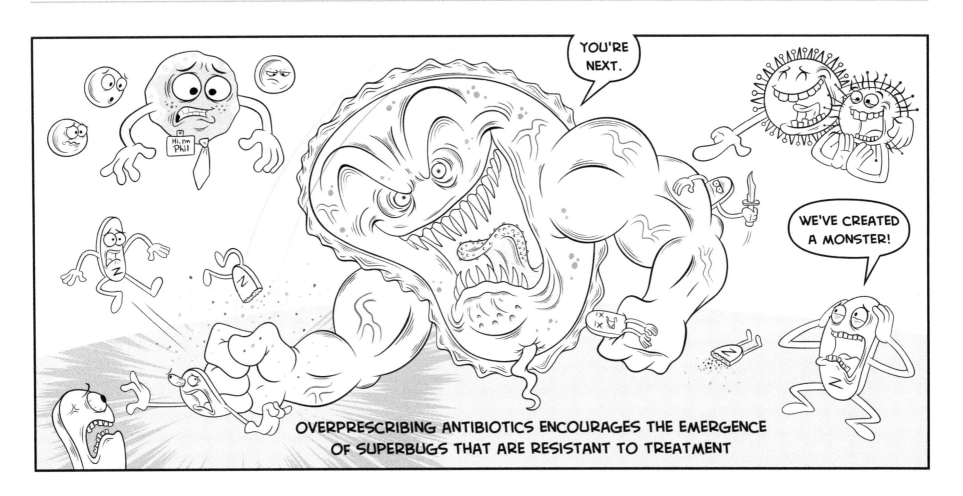

OTOLARYNGOLOGY

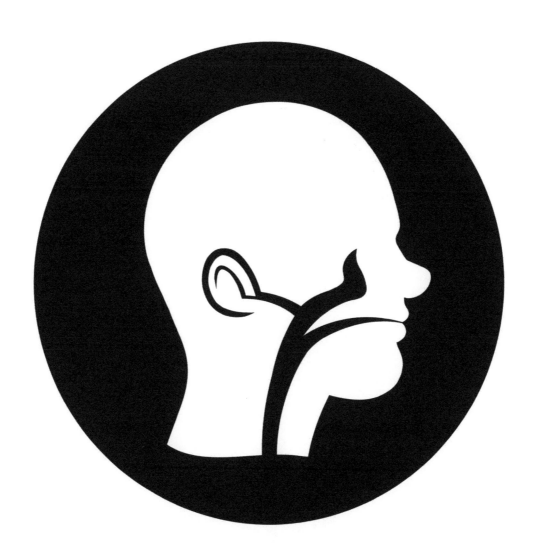

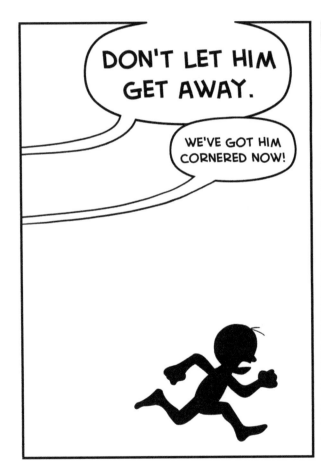

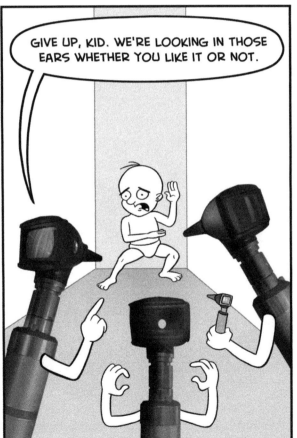

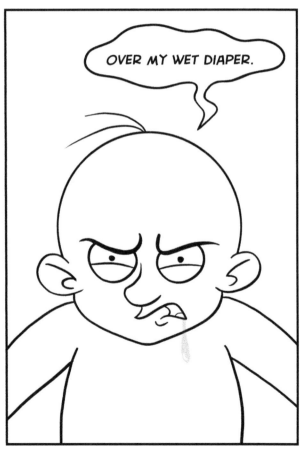

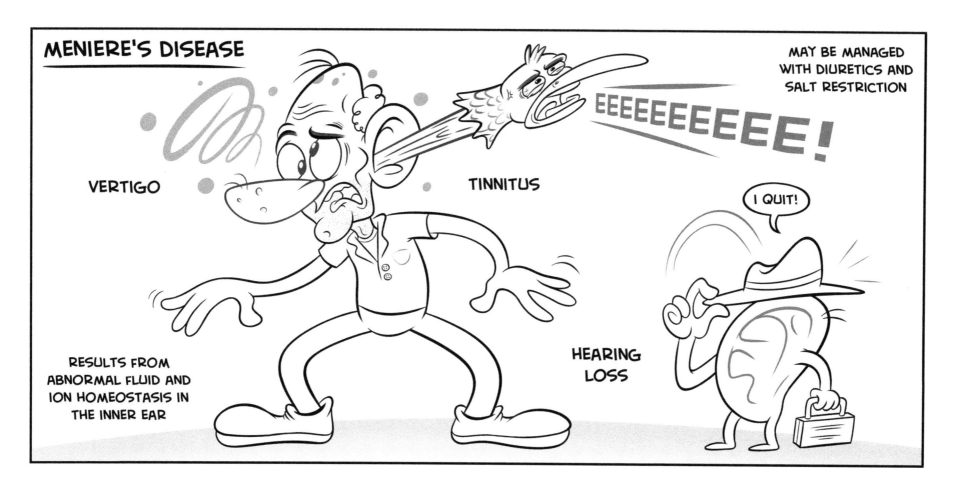

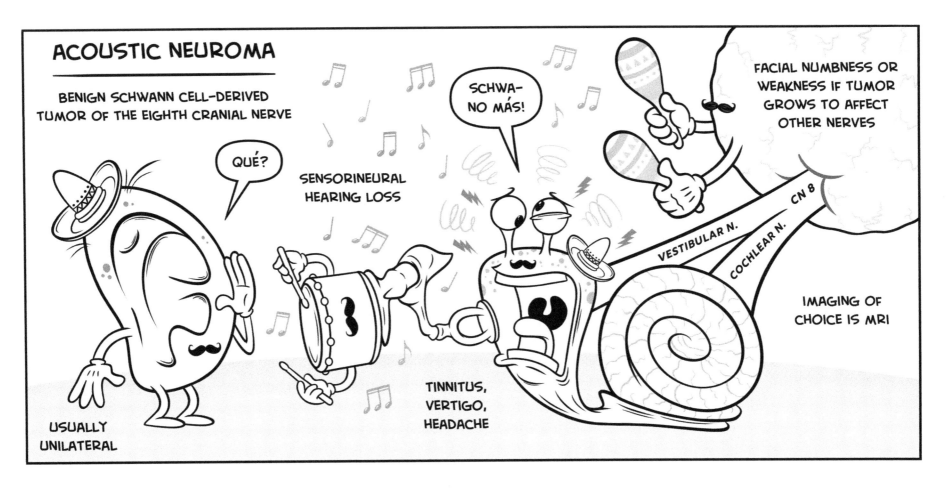

PERITONSILLAR ABSCESS

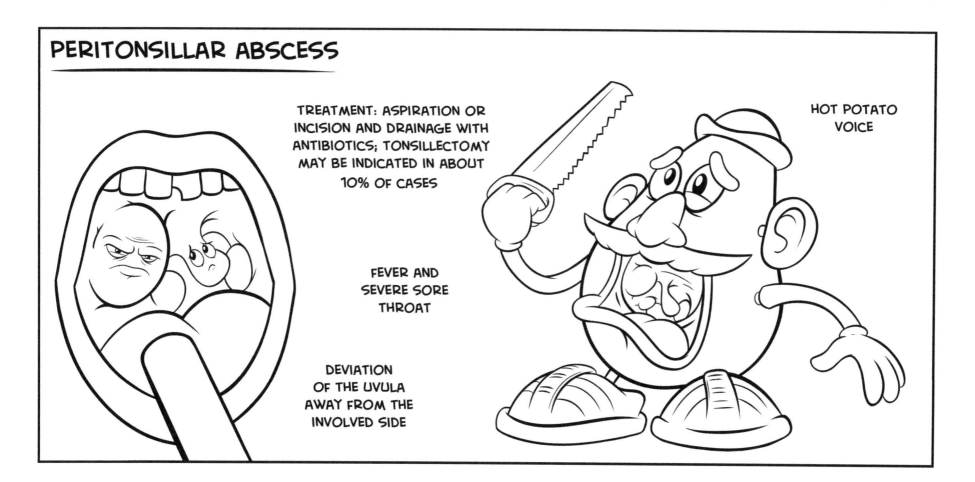

TREATMENT: ASPIRATION OR INCISION AND DRAINAGE WITH ANTIBIOTICS; TONSILLECTOMY MAY BE INDICATED IN ABOUT 10% OF CASES

HOT POTATO VOICE

FEVER AND SEVERE SORE THROAT

DEVIATION OF THE UVULA AWAY FROM THE INVOLVED SIDE

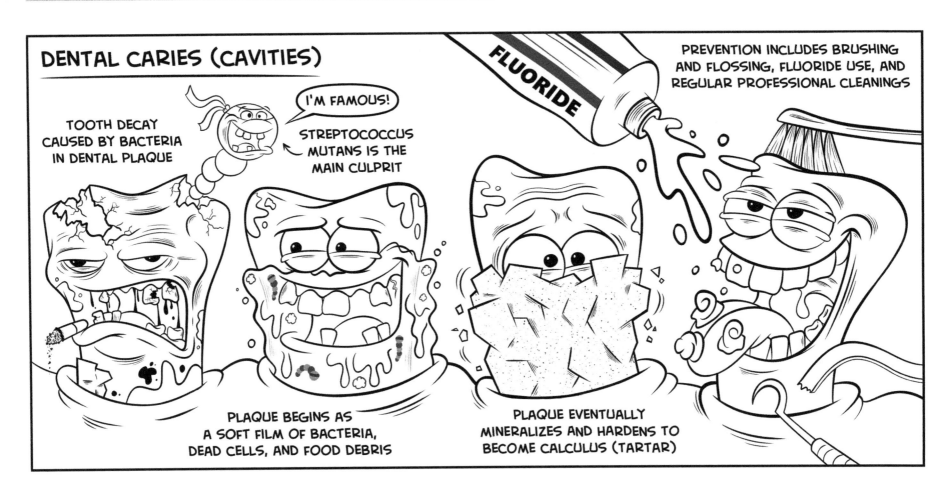

GASTROENTEROLOGY

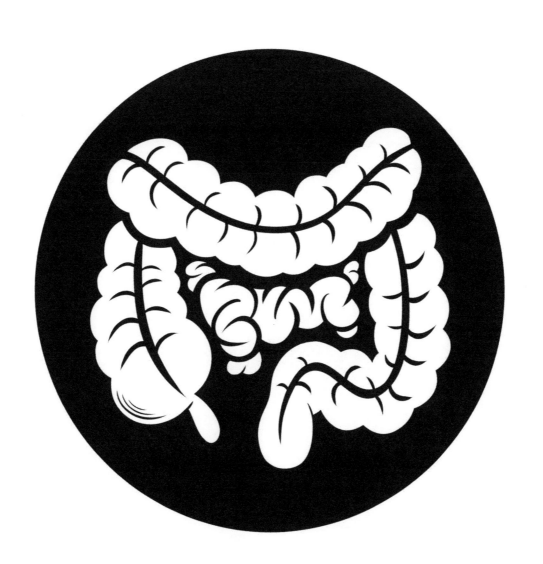

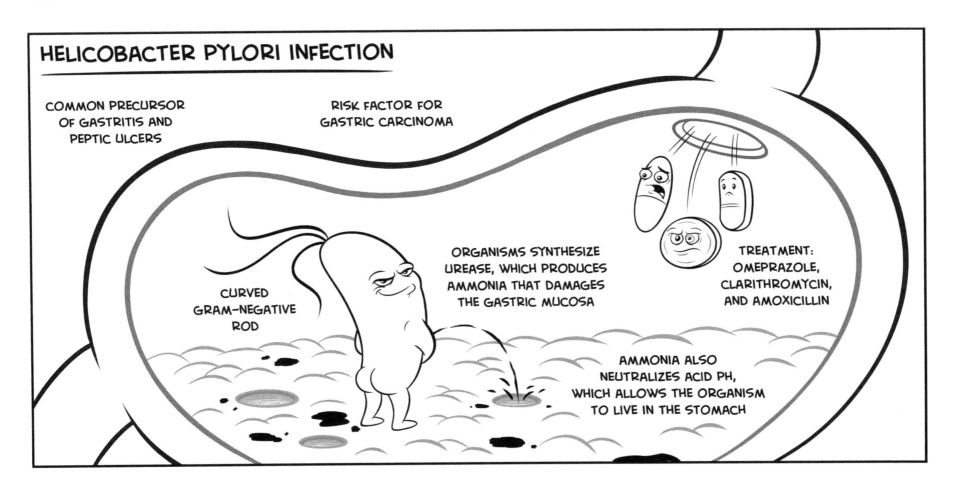

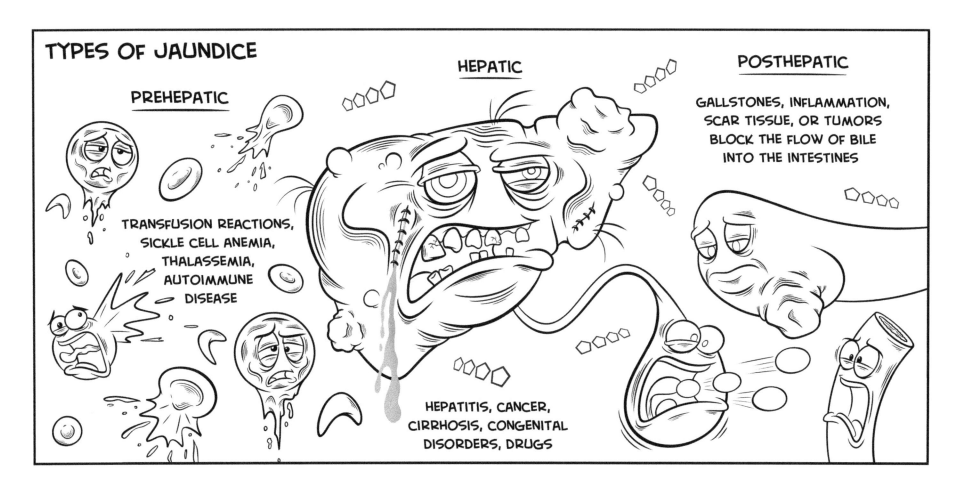

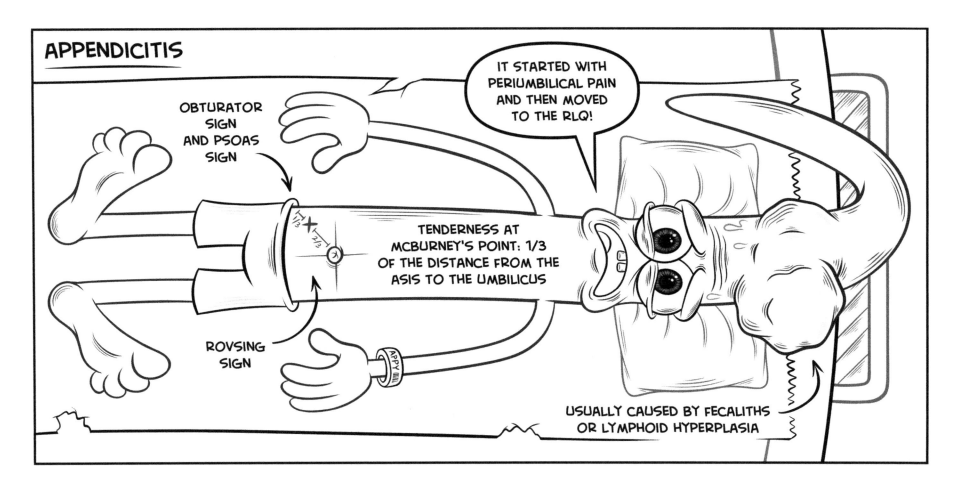

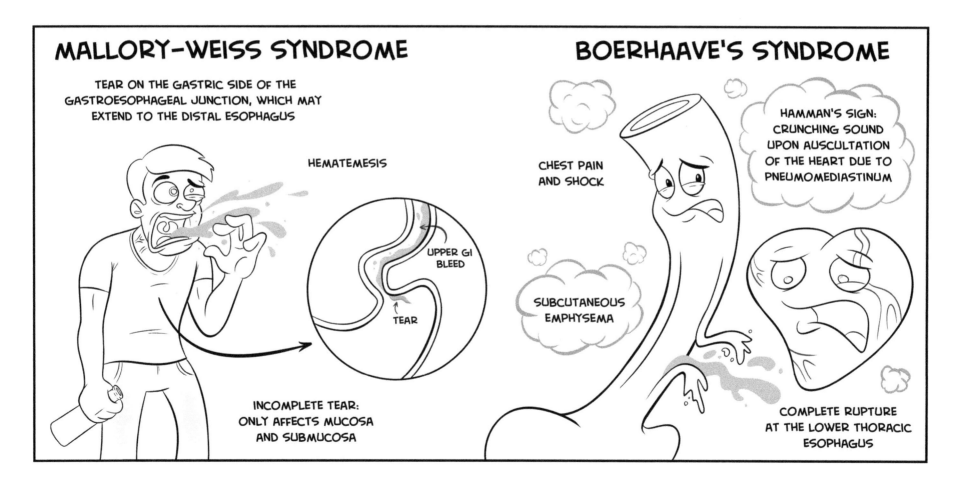

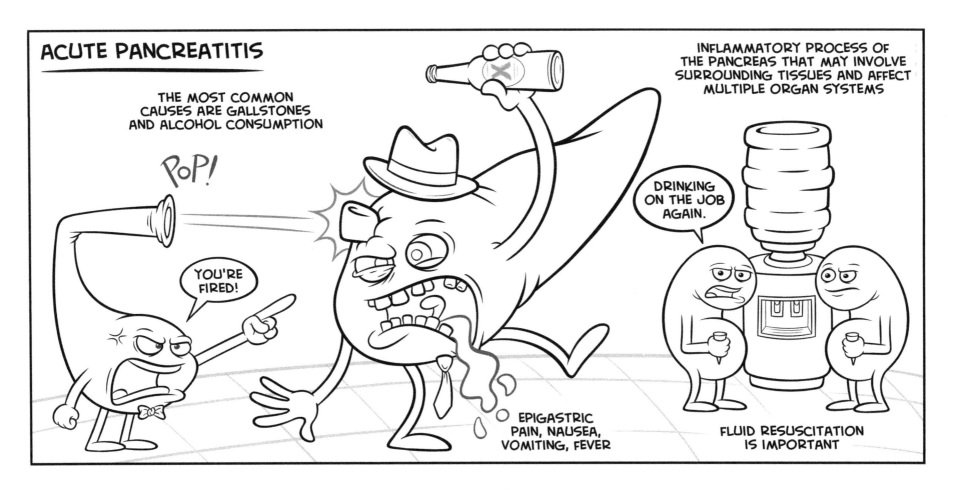

Ranson criteria present on admission	Ranson criteria present at 48 hours
A. Age > _____ years	**F.** Hematocrit fall of _____ % or greater
B. WBC > _____ /uL	**G.** BUN increase to > _____ mg/dL (> 1.98 mmol/L) despite fluids
C. Glucose > _____ (> 11 mmol/L)	**H.** Serum calcium < _____ mg/dL (< 2 mmol/L)
D. LDH > _____ IU/L	**I.** pO2 < _____ mmHg
E. AST > _____ IU/L	**J.** Base deficit > _____ meq/L (> 4 mmol/L)

HEPATITIS B INFECTION

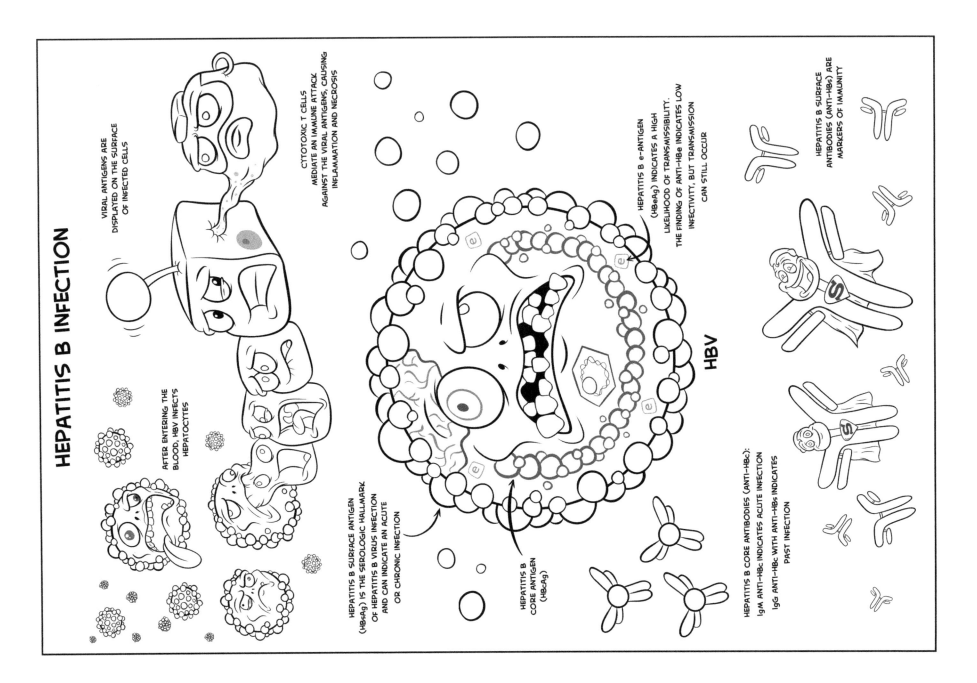

VIRAL ANTIGENS ARE DISPLAYED ON THE SURFACE OF INFECTED CELLS

CYTOTOXIC T CELLS MEDIATE AN IMMUNE ATTACK AGAINST THE VIRAL ANTIGENS, CAUSING INFLAMMATION AND NECROSIS

HEPATITIS B e-ANTIGEN (HBeAg) INDICATES A HIGH LIKELIHOOD OF TRANSMISSIBILITY. THE FINDING OF ANTI-HBe INDICATES LOW INFECTIVITY, BUT TRANSMISSION CAN STILL OCCUR

HEPATITIS B SURFACE ANTIBODIES (ANTI-HBs) ARE MARKERS OF IMMUNITY

AFTER ENTERING THE BLOOD, HBV INFECTS HEPATOCYTES

HEPATITIS B SURFACE ANTIGEN (HBsAg) IS THE SEROLOGIC HALLMARK OF HEPATITIS B VIRUS INFECTION AND CAN INDICATE AN ACUTE OR CHRONIC INFECTION

HEPATITIS B CORE ANTIGEN (HBcAg)

HEPATITIS B CORE ANTIBODIES (ANTI-HBc): IgM ANTI-HBc INDICATES ACUTE INFECTION IgG ANTI-HBc WITH ANTI-HBs INDICATES PAST INFECTION

HBV

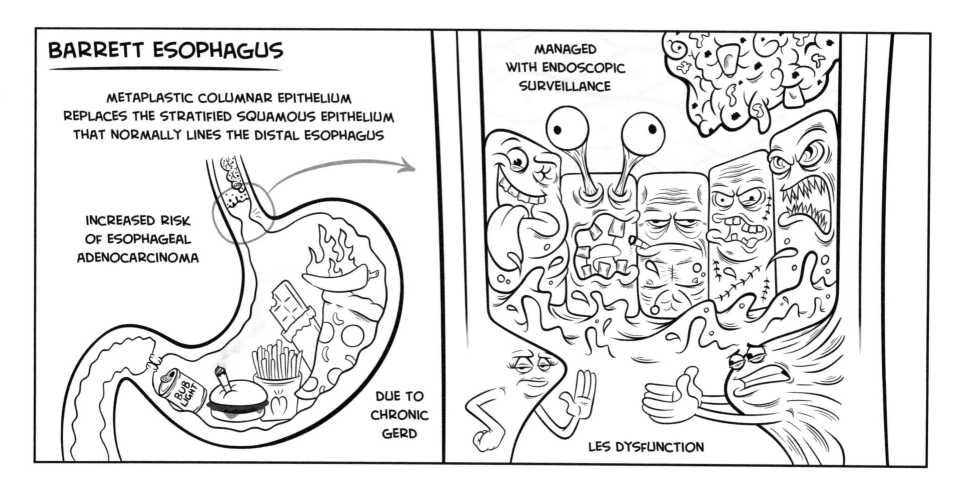

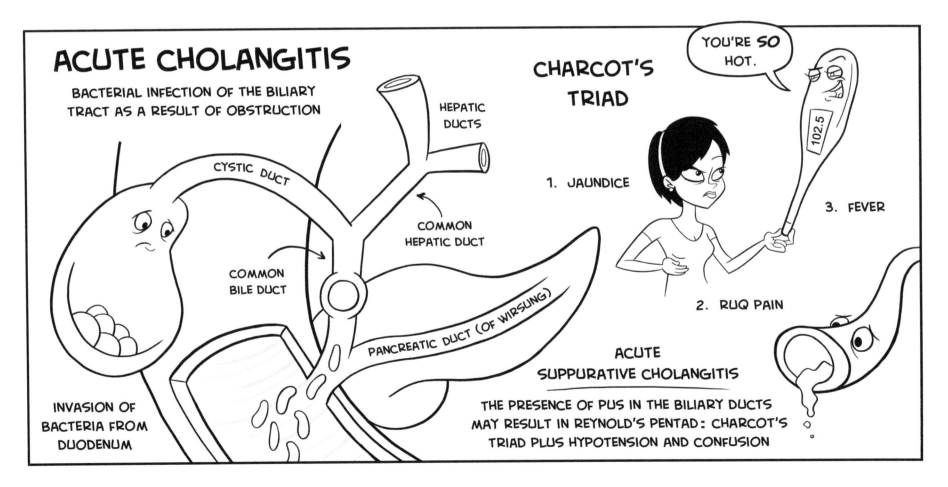

CROHN'S DISEASE

MAY INVOLVE ANY SEGMENT OF THE
GI TRACT FROM THE MOUTH TO THE ANUS

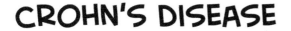

PROLONGED DIARRHEA WITH ABDOMINAL
PAIN, FATIGUE, & WEIGHT LOSS

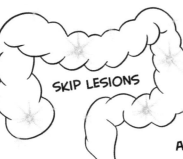

SKIP LESIONS

TRANSMURAL
INFLAMMATION

ANAL FISTULAE,
ABSCESSES,
FISSURES, AND ULCERS

EXTRAINTESTINAL
MANIFESTATIONS OF IBD

ORAL ULCERS
ARTHRITIS
SPONDYLITIS OR SACROILIITIS
EPISCLERITIS OR UVEITIS
ERYTHEMA NODOSUM
PYODERMA GANGRENOSUM
HEPATITIS
SCLEROSING CHOLANGITIS
THROMBOEMBOLIC EVENTS

ULCERATIVE COLITIS

RECURRING EPISODES OF INFLAMMATION
LIMITED TO THE MUCOSAL LAYER
OF THE COLON

BLOODY
DIARRHEA
WITH MUCUS

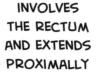

INVOLVES
THE RECTUM
AND EXTENDS
PROXIMALLY

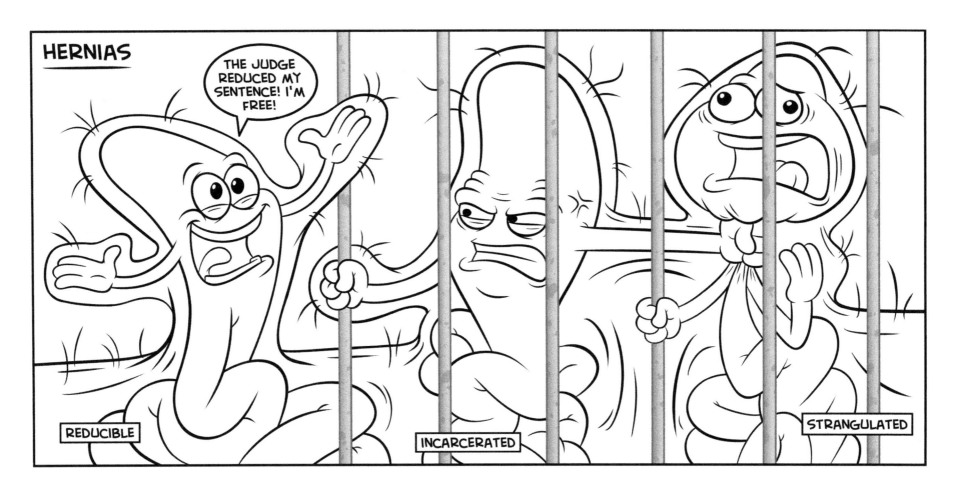

PEDIATRICS

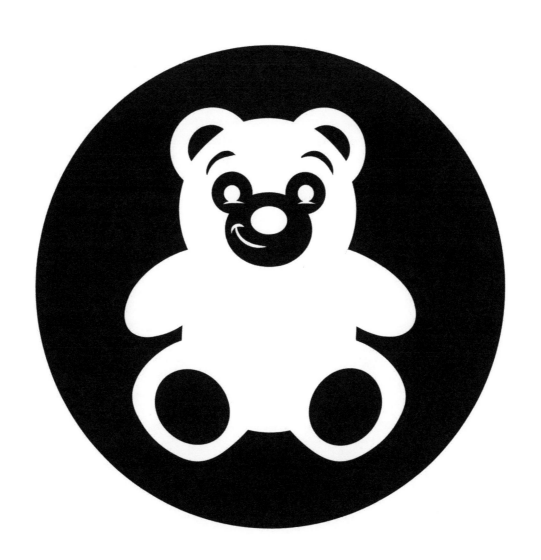

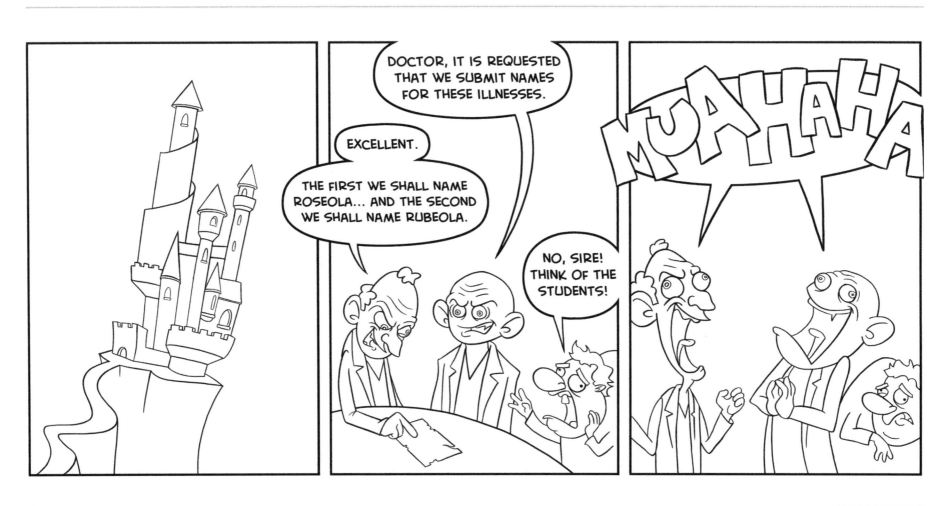

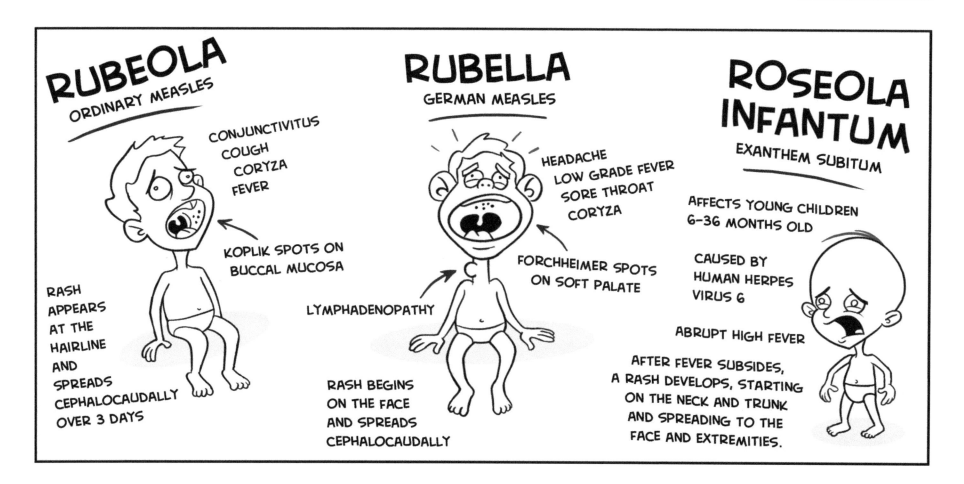

RUBEOLA
ORDINARY MEASLES

CONJUNCTIVITUS
COUGH
CORYZA
FEVER

KOPLIK SPOTS ON
BUCCAL MUCOSA

RASH
APPEARS
AT THE
HAIRLINE
AND
SPREADS
CEPHALOCAUDALLY
OVER 3 DAYS

RUBELLA
GERMAN MEASLES

HEADACHE
LOW GRADE FEVER
SORE THROAT
CORYZA

FORCHHEIMER SPOTS
ON SOFT PALATE

LYMPHADENOPATHY

RASH BEGINS
ON THE FACE
AND SPREADS
CEPHALOCAUDALLY

ROSEOLA INFANTUM
EXANTHEM SUBITUM

AFFECTS YOUNG CHILDREN
6-36 MONTHS OLD

CAUSED BY
HUMAN HERPES
VIRUS 6

ABRUPT HIGH FEVER

AFTER FEVER SUBSIDES,
A RASH DEVELOPS, STARTING
ON THE NECK AND TRUNK
AND SPREADING TO THE
FACE AND EXTREMITIES.

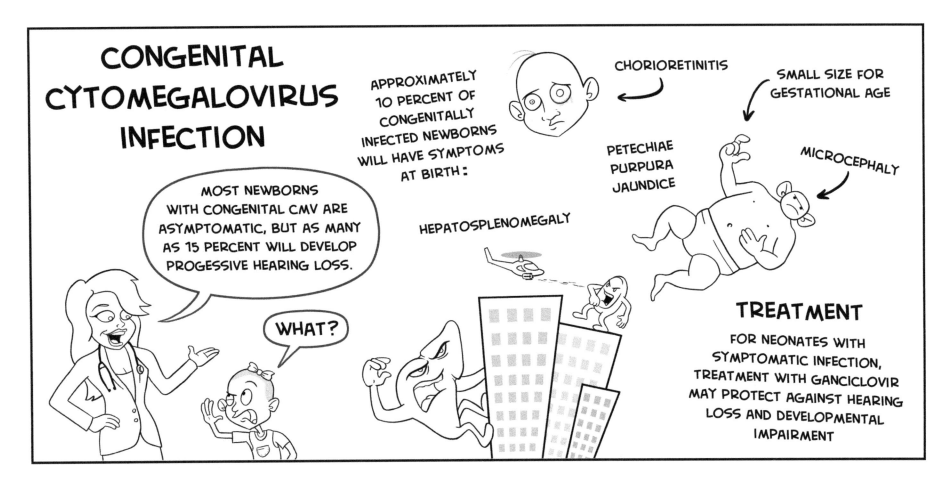

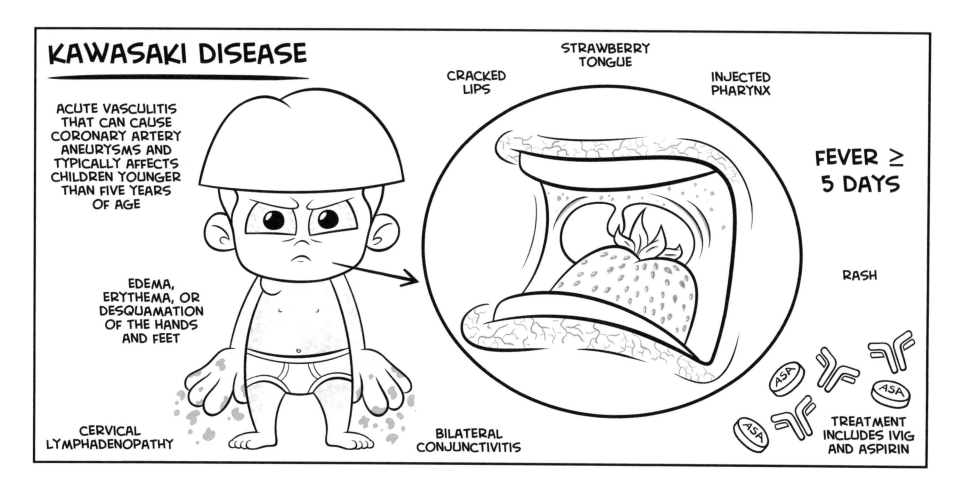

KAWASAKI DISEASE

ACUTE VASCULITIS THAT CAN CAUSE CORONARY ARTERY ANEURYSMS AND TYPICALLY AFFECTS CHILDREN YOUNGER THAN FIVE YEARS OF AGE

EDEMA, ERYTHEMA, OR DESQUAMATION OF THE HANDS AND FEET

CERVICAL LYMPHADENOPATHY

CRACKED LIPS

STRAWBERRY TONGUE

INJECTED PHARYNX

FEVER ≥ 5 DAYS

RASH

BILATERAL CONJUNCTIVITIS

TREATMENT INCLUDES IVIG AND ASPIRIN

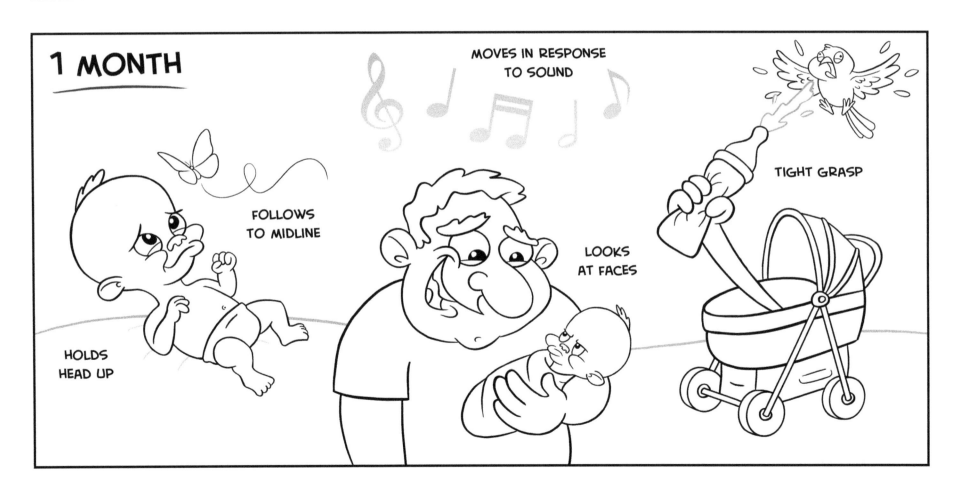

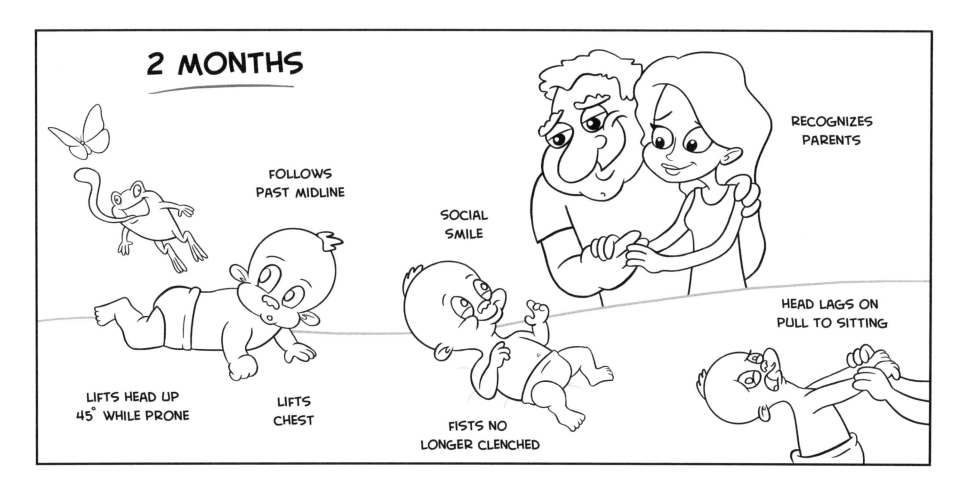

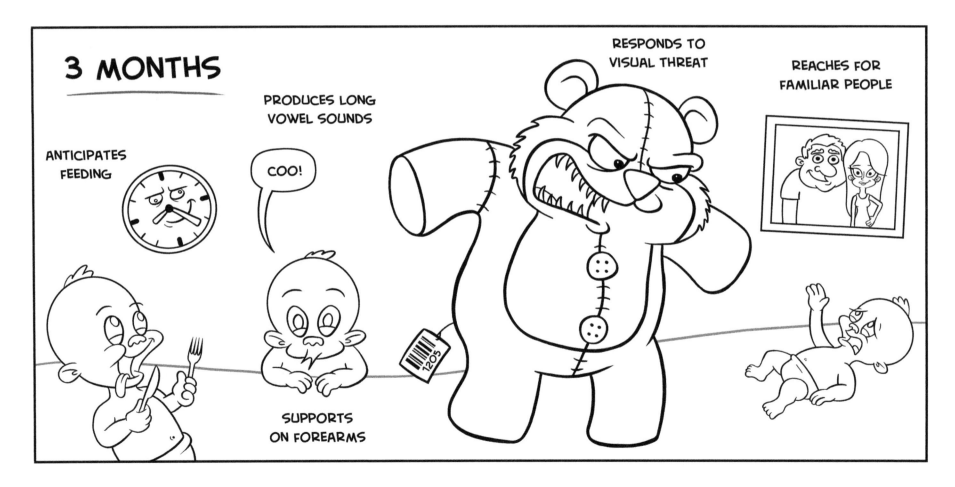

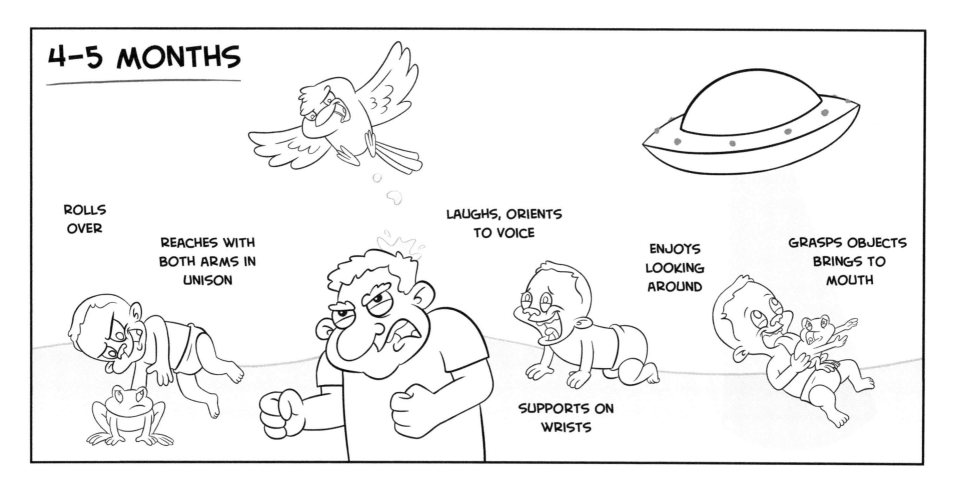

4-5 MONTHS

ROLLS OVER

REACHES WITH BOTH ARMS IN UNISON

LAUGHS, ORIENTS TO VOICE

ENJOYS LOOKING AROUND

GRASPS OBJECTS BRINGS TO MOUTH

SUPPORTS ON WRISTS

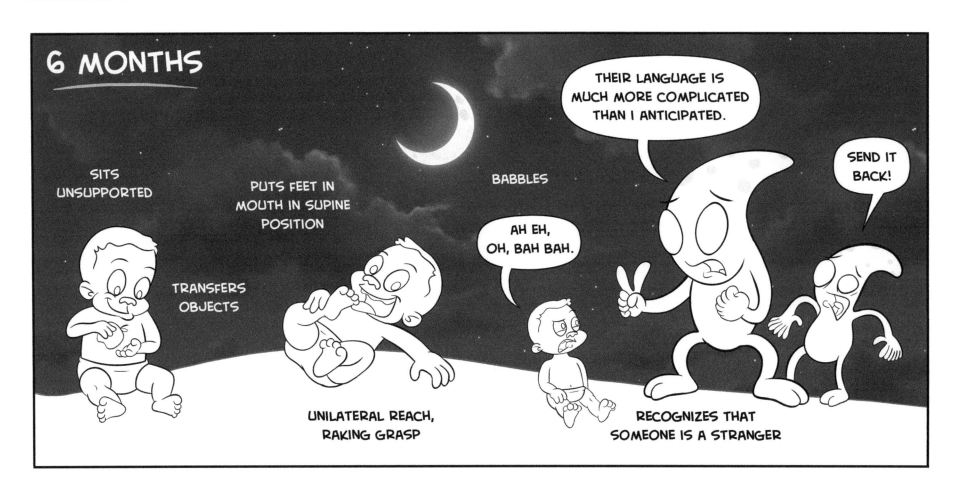

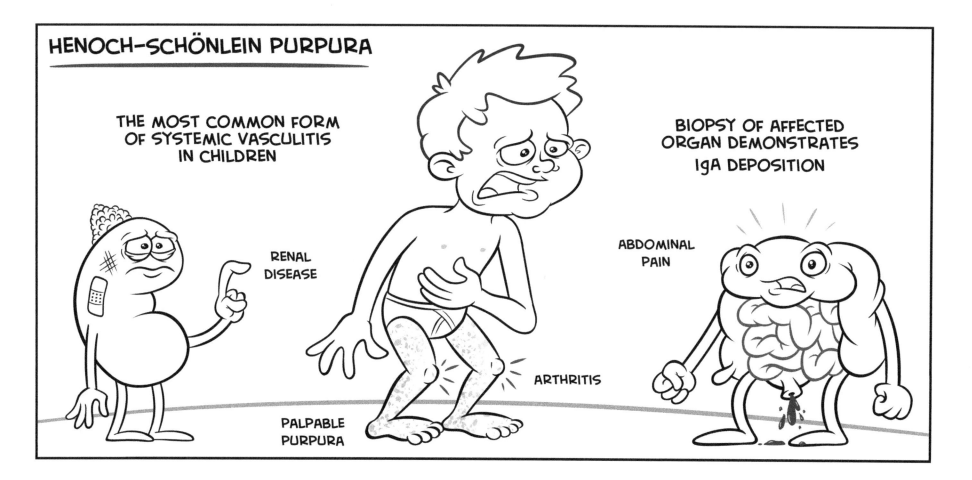

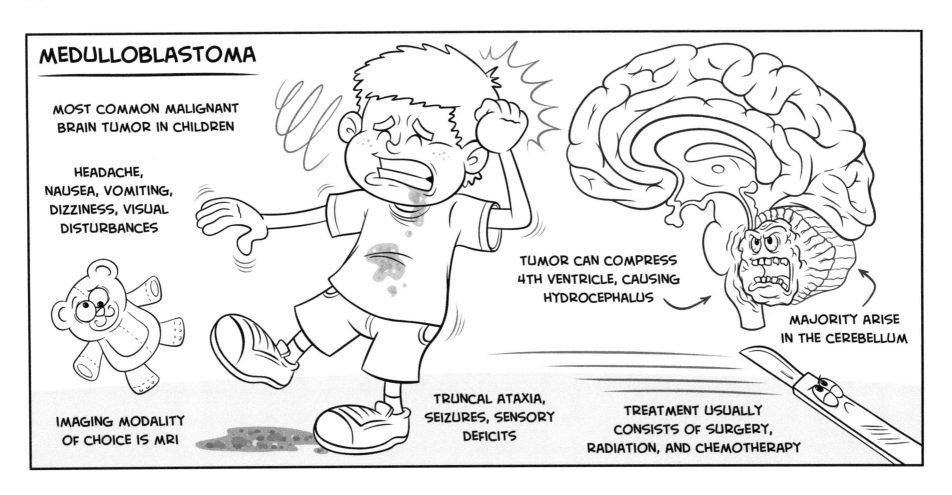

MEDULLOBLASTOMA

MOST COMMON MALIGNANT BRAIN TUMOR IN CHILDREN

HEADACHE, NAUSEA, VOMITING, DIZZINESS, VISUAL DISTURBANCES

IMAGING MODALITY OF CHOICE IS MRI

TUMOR CAN COMPRESS 4TH VENTRICLE, CAUSING HYDROCEPHALUS

MAJORITY ARISE IN THE CEREBELLUM

TRUNCAL ATAXIA, SEIZURES, SENSORY DEFICITS

TREATMENT USUALLY CONSISTS OF SURGERY, RADIATION, AND CHEMOTHERAPY

NEPHROLOGY AND UROLOGY

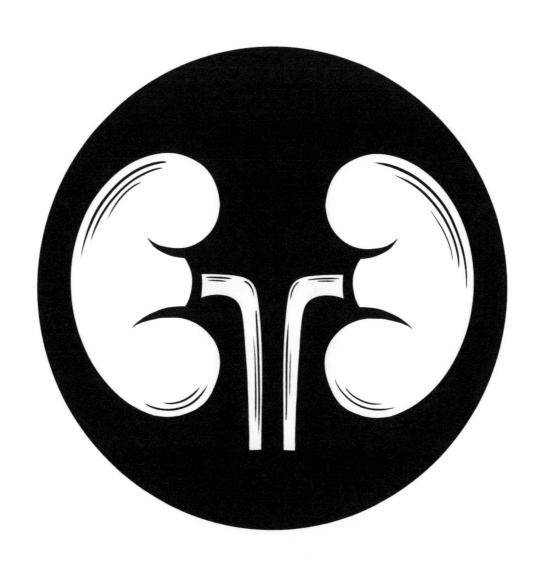

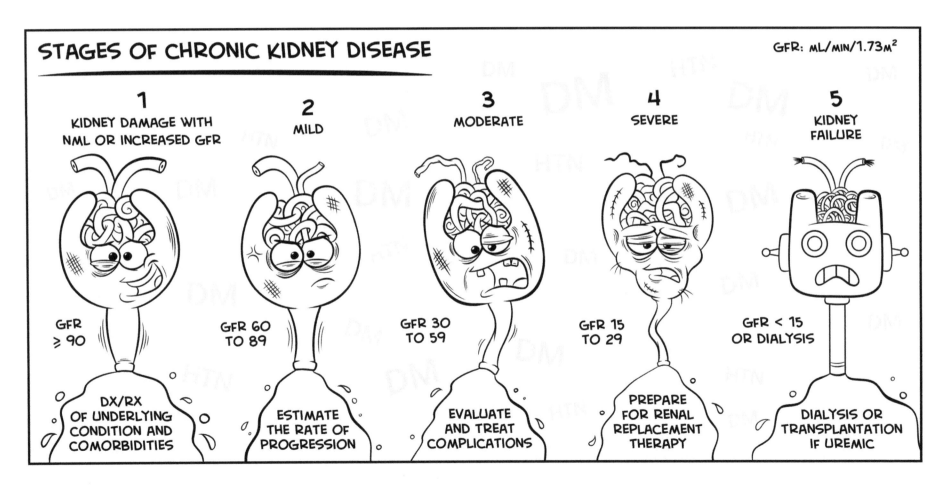

STAGES OF CHRONIC KIDNEY DISEASE

GFR: ML/MIN/1.73M²

1
KIDNEY DAMAGE WITH
NML OR INCREASED GFR

GFR ≥ 90

DX/RX
OF UNDERLYING
CONDITION AND
COMORBIDITIES

2
MILD

GFR 60
TO 89

ESTIMATE
THE RATE OF
PROGRESSION

3
MODERATE

GFR 30
TO 59

EVALUATE
AND TREAT
COMPLICATIONS

4
SEVERE

GFR 15
TO 29

PREPARE
FOR RENAL
REPLACEMENT
THERAPY

5
KIDNEY
FAILURE

GFR < 15
OR DIALYSIS

DIALYSIS OR
TRANSPLANTATION
IF UREMIC

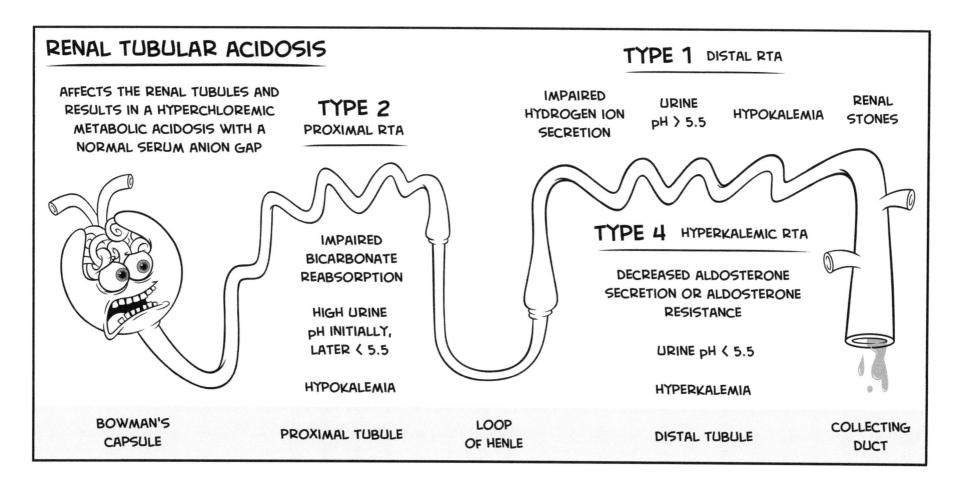

RENAL TUBULAR ACIDOSIS

AFFECTS THE RENAL TUBULES AND RESULTS IN A HYPERCHLOREMIC METABOLIC ACIDOSIS WITH A NORMAL SERUM ANION GAP

TYPE 2 PROXIMAL RTA

IMPAIRED BICARBONATE REABSORPTION

HIGH URINE pH INITIALLY, LATER < 5.5

HYPOKALEMIA

TYPE 1 DISTAL RTA

IMPAIRED HYDROGEN ION SECRETION

URINE pH > 5.5

HYPOKALEMIA

RENAL STONES

TYPE 4 HYPERKALEMIC RTA

DECREASED ALDOSTERONE SECRETION OR ALDOSTERONE RESISTANCE

URINE pH < 5.5

HYPERKALEMIA

BOWMAN'S CAPSULE

PROXIMAL TUBULE

LOOP OF HENLE

DISTAL TUBULE

COLLECTING DUCT

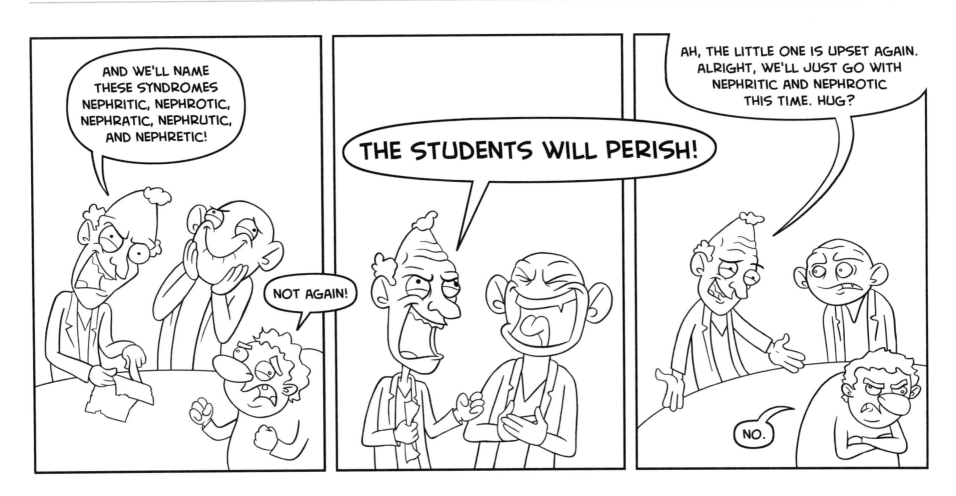

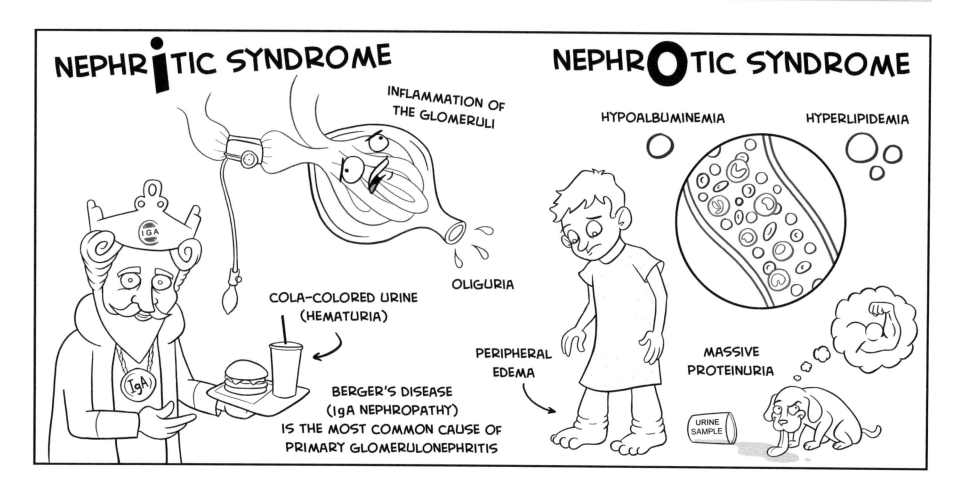

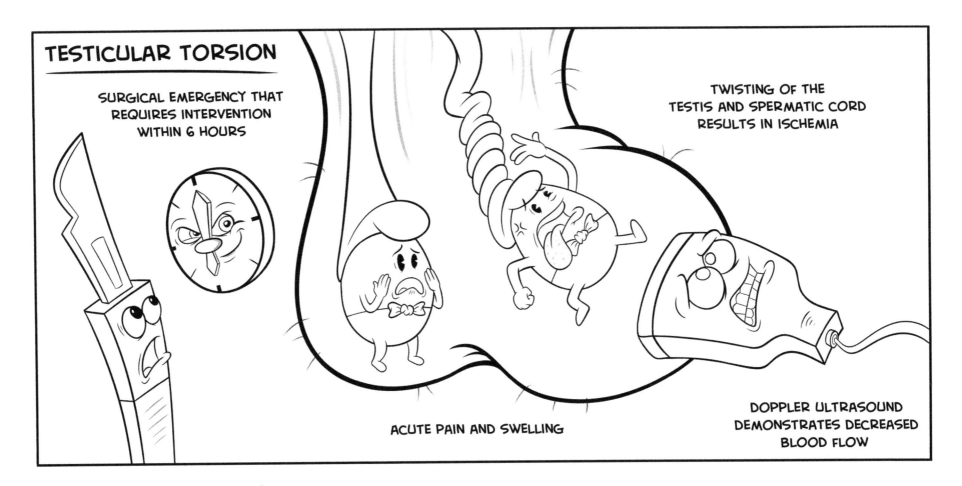

TESTICULAR TORSION

SURGICAL EMERGENCY THAT REQUIRES INTERVENTION WITHIN 6 HOURS

TWISTING OF THE TESTIS AND SPERMATIC CORD RESULTS IN ISCHEMIA

ACUTE PAIN AND SWELLING

DOPPLER ULTRASOUND DEMONSTRATES DECREASED BLOOD FLOW

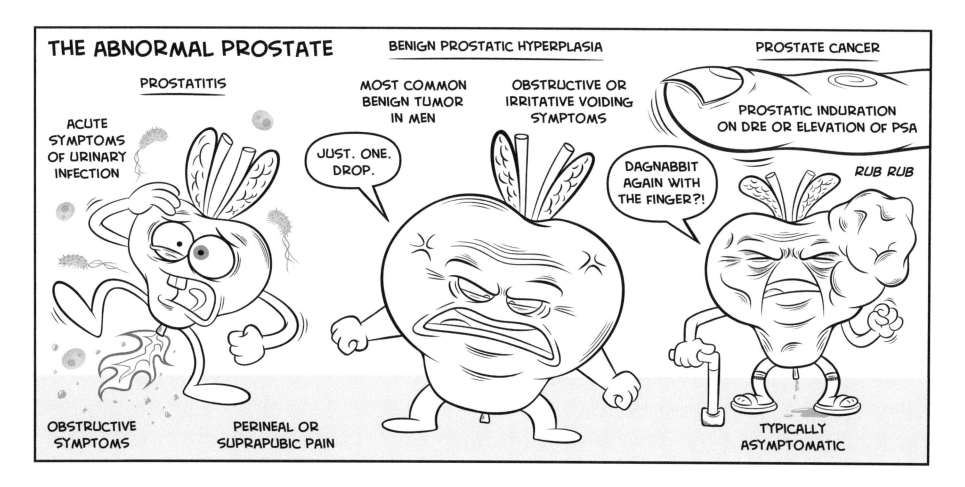

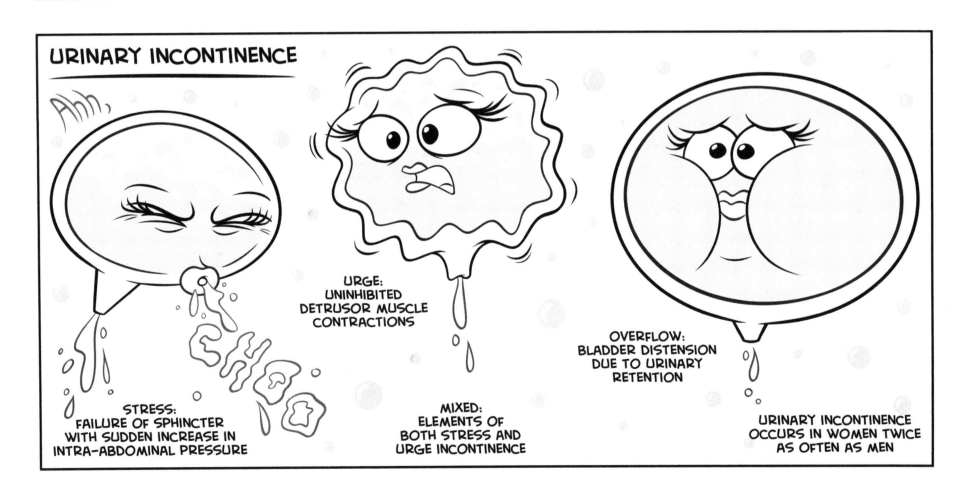

OPHTHALMOLOGY

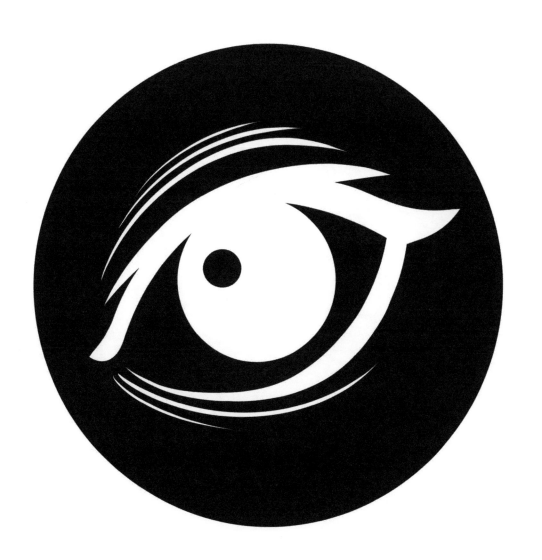

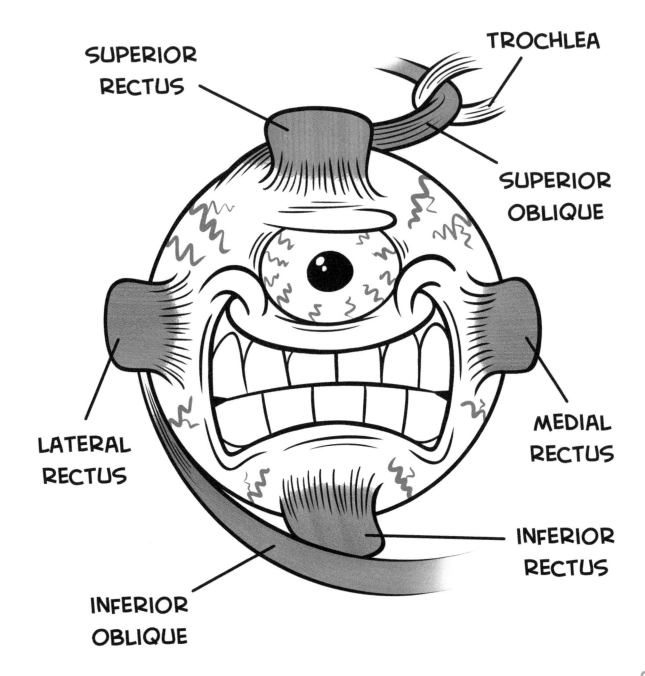

SUPERIOR
RECTUS

TROCHLEA

SUPERIOR
OBLIQUE

MEDIAL
RECTUS

INFERIOR
RECTUS

INFERIOR
OBLIQUE

LATERAL
RECTUS

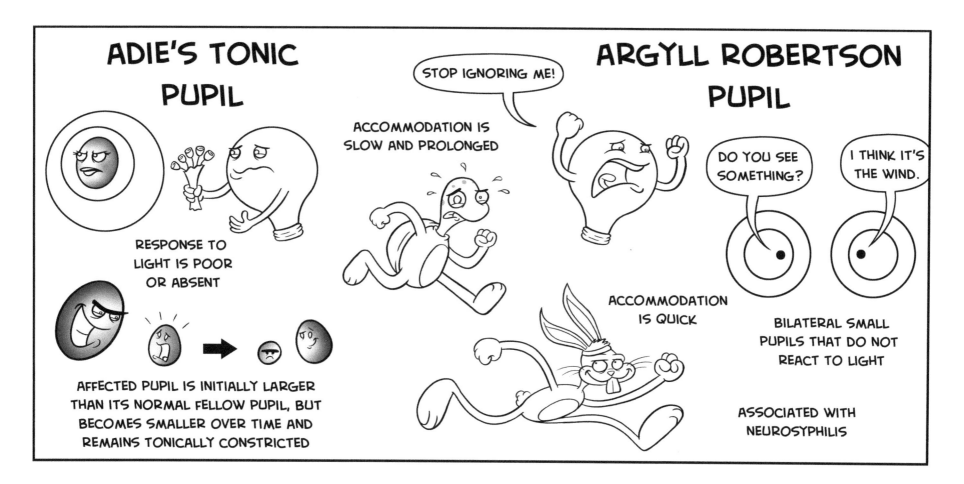

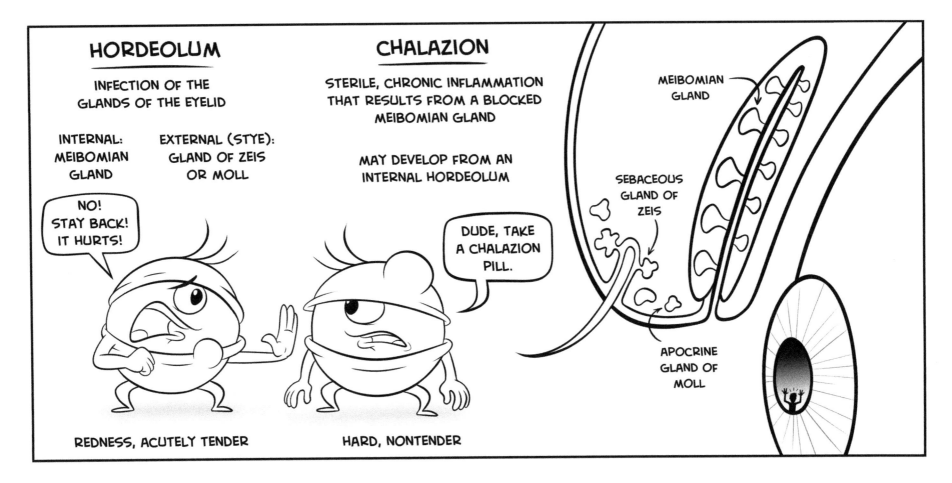

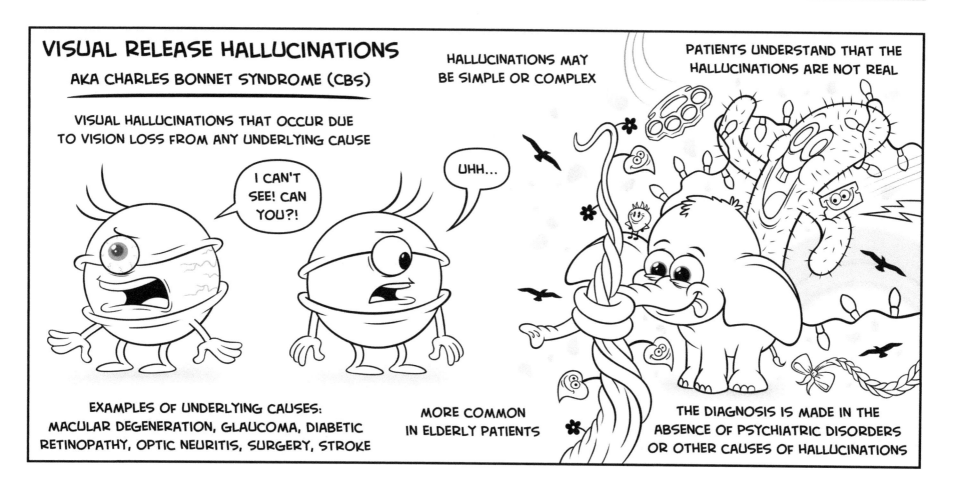

VISUAL RELEASE HALLUCINATIONS
AKA CHARLES BONNET SYNDROME (CBS)

VISUAL HALLUCINATIONS THAT OCCUR DUE TO VISION LOSS FROM ANY UNDERLYING CAUSE

EXAMPLES OF UNDERLYING CAUSES: MACULAR DEGENERATION, GLAUCOMA, DIABETIC RETINOPATHY, OPTIC NEURITIS, SURGERY, STROKE

HALLUCINATIONS MAY BE SIMPLE OR COMPLEX

MORE COMMON IN ELDERLY PATIENTS

PATIENTS UNDERSTAND THAT THE HALLUCINATIONS ARE NOT REAL

THE DIAGNOSIS IS MADE IN THE ABSENCE OF PSYCHIATRIC DISORDERS OR OTHER CAUSES OF HALLUCINATIONS

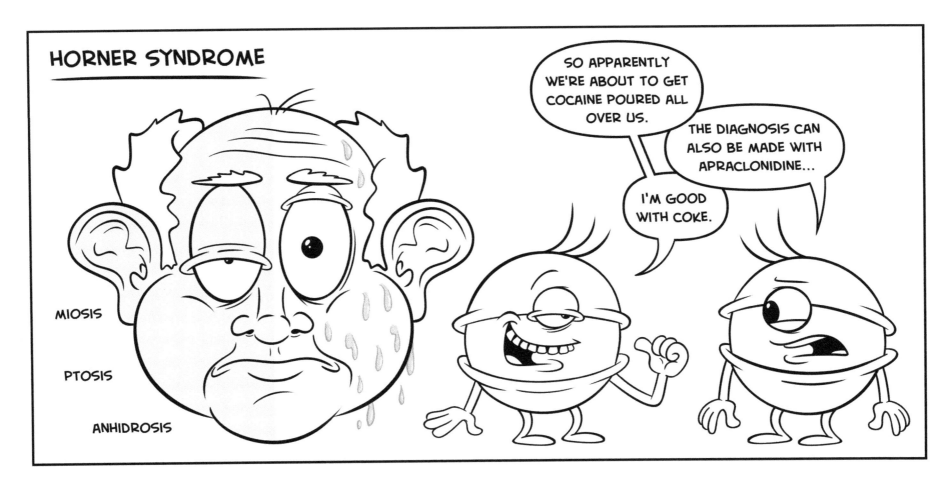

OBSTETRICS AND GYNECOLOGY

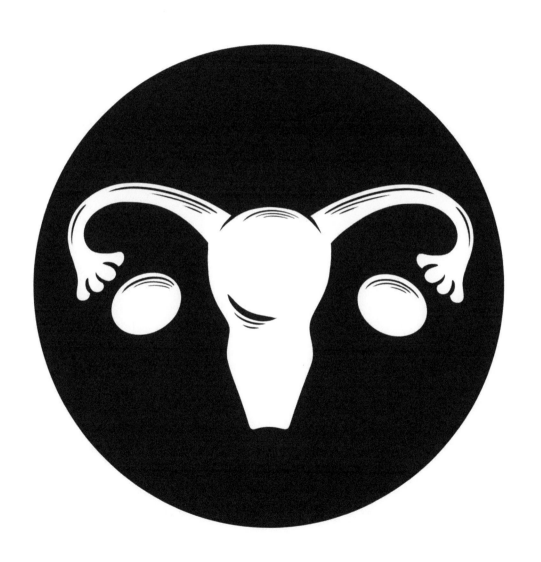

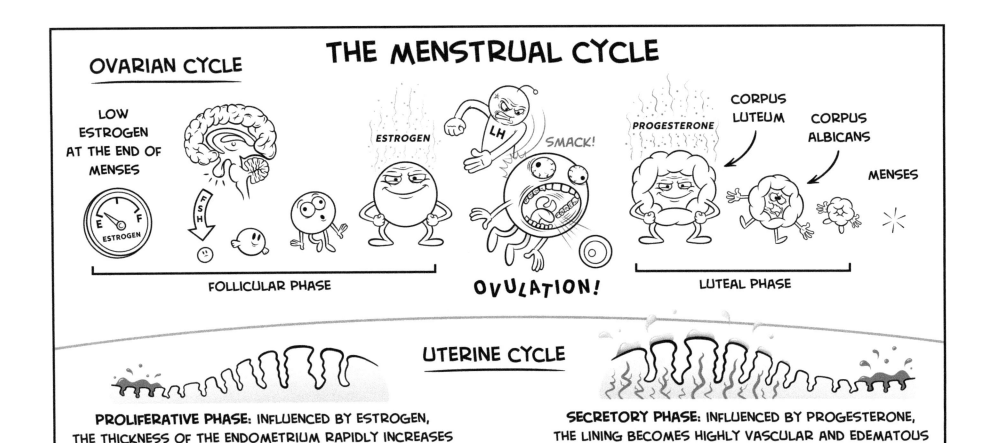

THE MENSTRUAL CYCLE

OVARIAN CYCLE

LOW ESTROGEN AT THE END OF MENSES

ESTROGEN

SMACK!

LH

PROGESTERONE

CORPUS LUTEUM

CORPUS ALBICANS

MENSES

FOLLICULAR PHASE

OVULATION!

LUTEAL PHASE

UTERINE CYCLE

PROLIFERATIVE PHASE: INFLUENCED BY ESTROGEN, THE THICKNESS OF THE ENDOMETRIUM RAPIDLY INCREASES

SECRETORY PHASE: INFLUENCED BY PROGESTERONE, THE LINING BECOMES HIGHLY VASCULAR AND EDEMATOUS

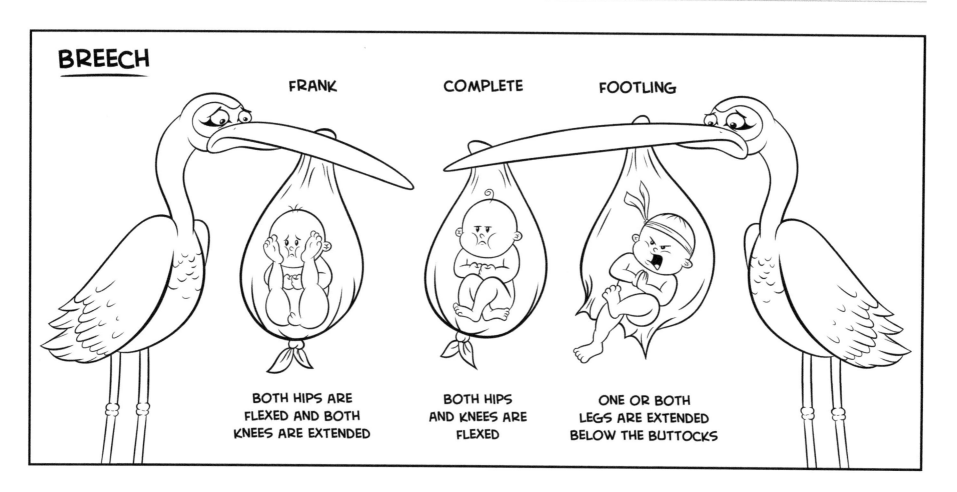

BREECH

FRANK

COMPLETE

FOOTLING

BOTH HIPS ARE
FLEXED AND BOTH
KNEES ARE EXTENDED

BOTH HIPS
AND KNEES ARE
FLEXED

ONE OR BOTH
LEGS ARE EXTENDED
BELOW THE BUTTOCKS

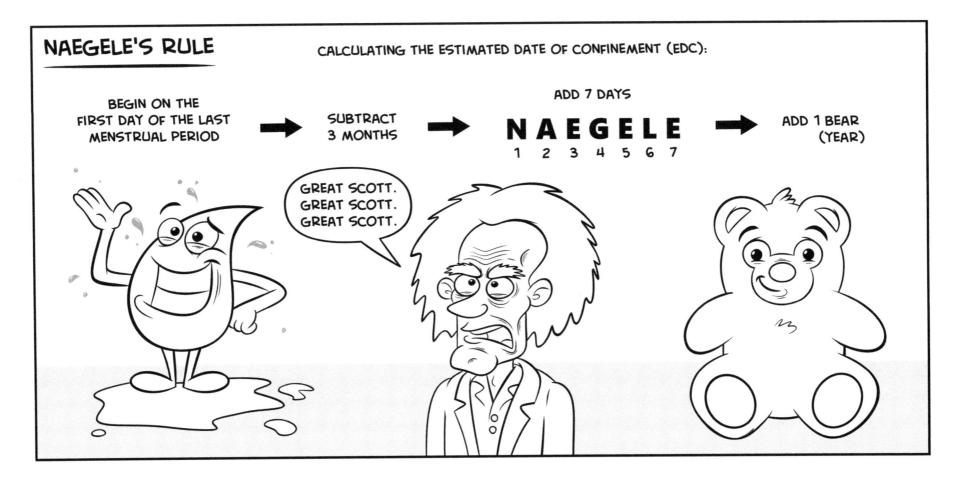

POLYCYSTIC OVARIAN SYNDROME

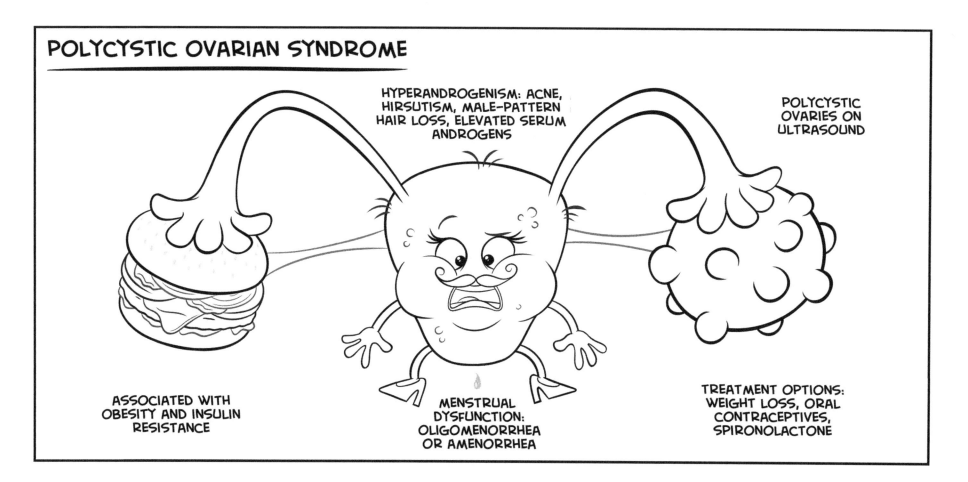

HYPERANDROGENISM: ACNE, HIRSUTISM, MALE-PATTERN HAIR LOSS, ELEVATED SERUM ANDROGENS

POLYCYSTIC OVARIES ON ULTRASOUND

ASSOCIATED WITH OBESITY AND INSULIN RESISTANCE

MENSTRUAL DYSFUNCTION: OLIGOMENORRHEA OR AMENORRHEA

TREATMENT OPTIONS: WEIGHT LOSS, ORAL CONTRACEPTIVES, SPIRONOLACTONE

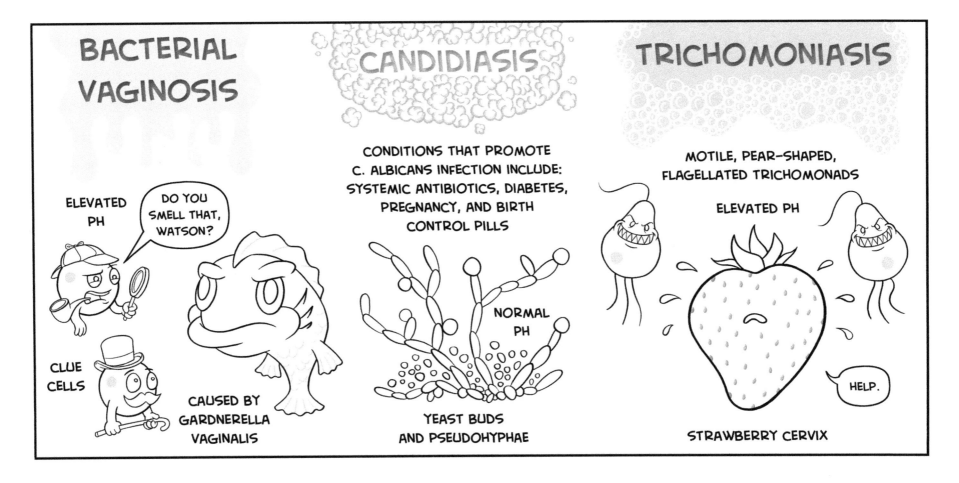

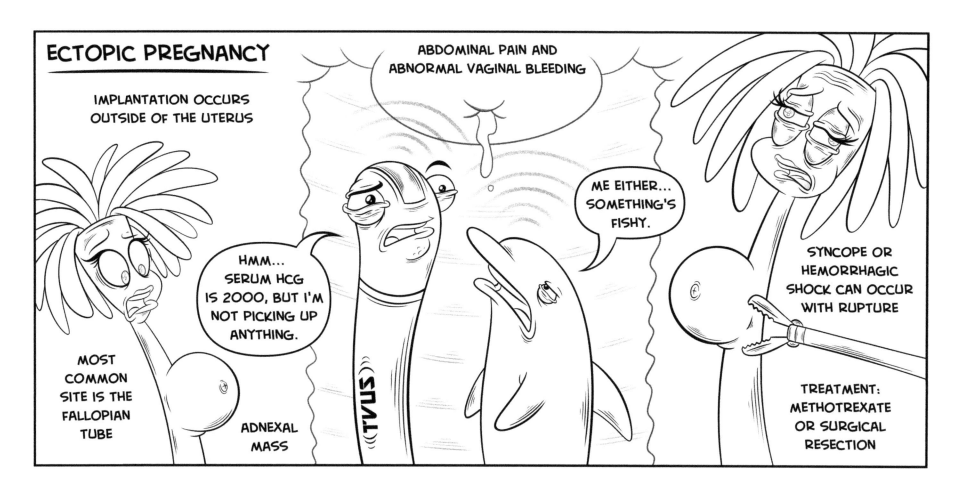

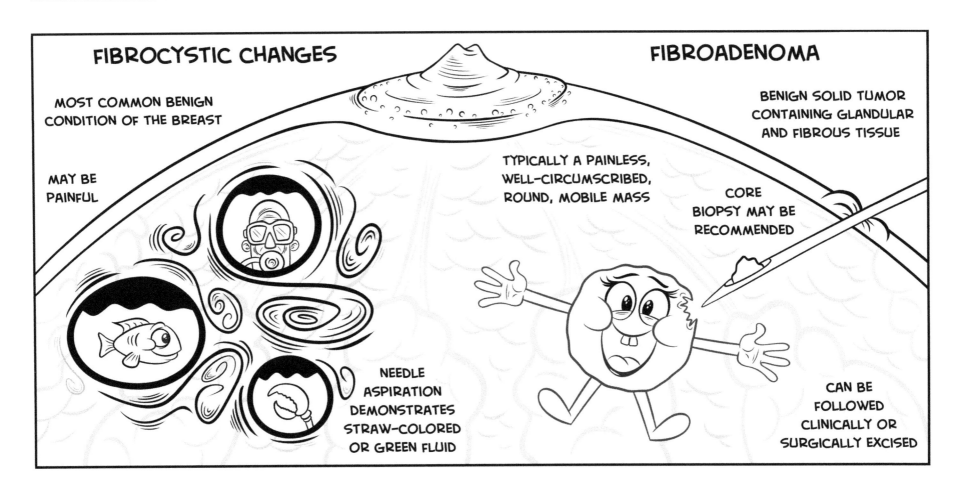

FIBROCYSTIC CHANGES

FIBROADENOMA

MOST COMMON BENIGN
CONDITION OF THE BREAST

MAY BE
PAINFUL

BENIGN SOLID TUMOR
CONTAINING GLANDULAR
AND FIBROUS TISSUE

TYPICALLY A PAINLESS,
WELL-CIRCUMSCRIBED,
ROUND, MOBILE MASS

CORE
BIOPSY MAY BE
RECOMMENDED

NEEDLE
ASPIRATION
DEMONSTRATES
STRAW-COLORED
OR GREEN FLUID

CAN BE
FOLLOWED
CLINICALLY OR
SURGICALLY EXCISED

DERMATOLOGY

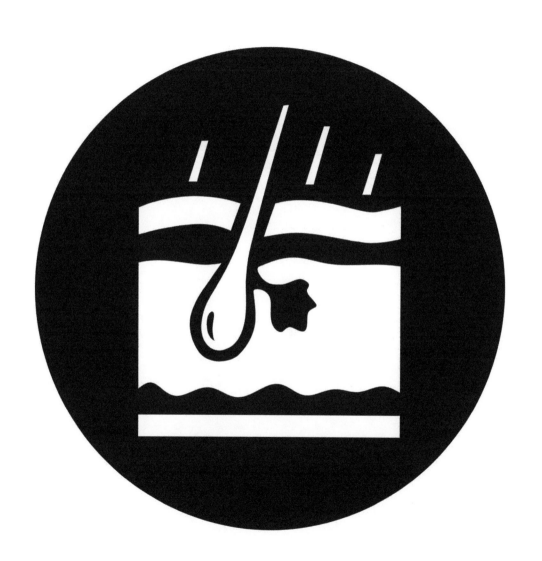

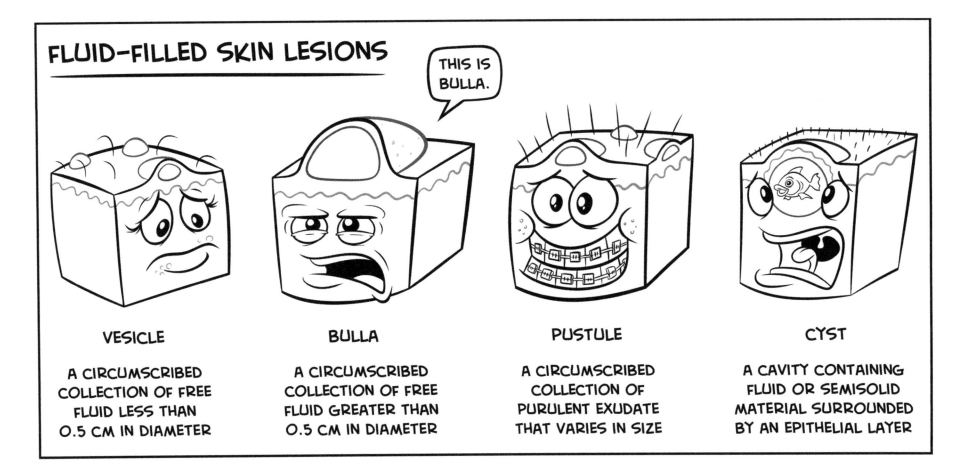

FLUID-FILLED SKIN LESIONS

THIS IS BULLA.

VESICLE

A CIRCUMSCRIBED COLLECTION OF FREE FLUID LESS THAN 0.5 CM IN DIAMETER

BULLA

A CIRCUMSCRIBED COLLECTION OF FREE FLUID GREATER THAN 0.5 CM IN DIAMETER

PUSTULE

A CIRCUMSCRIBED COLLECTION OF PURULENT EXUDATE THAT VARIES IN SIZE

CYST

A CAVITY CONTAINING FLUID OR SEMISOLID MATERIAL SURROUNDED BY AN EPITHELIAL LAYER

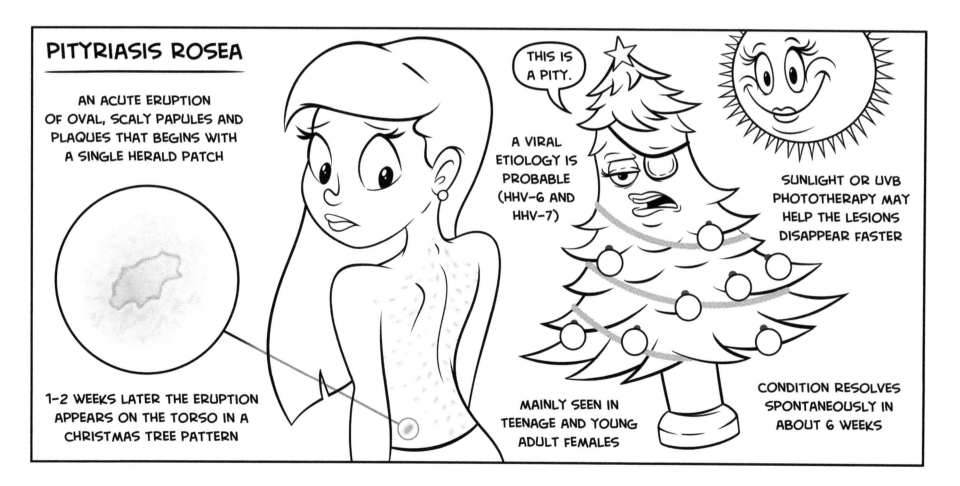

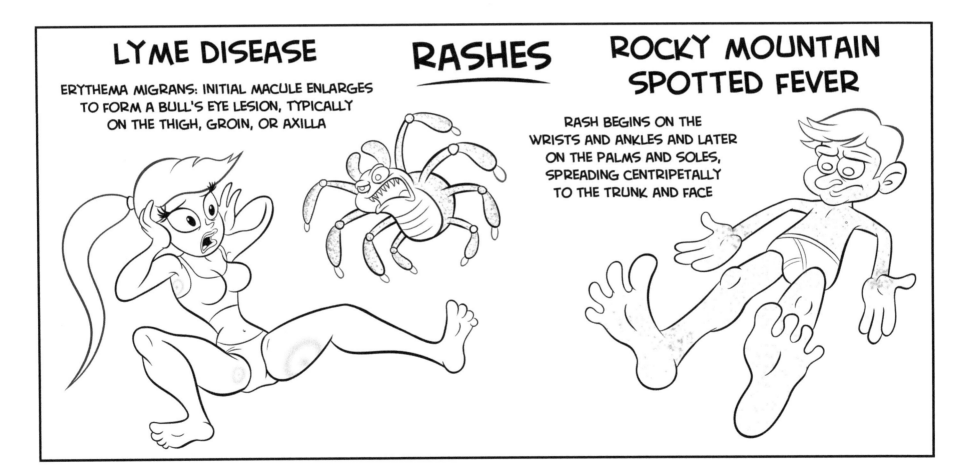

RASHES

LYME DISEASE

ERYTHEMA MIGRANS: INITIAL MACULE ENLARGES TO FORM A BULL'S EYE LESION, TYPICALLY ON THE THIGH, GROIN, OR AXILLA

ROCKY MOUNTAIN SPOTTED FEVER

RASH BEGINS ON THE WRISTS AND ANKLES AND LATER ON THE PALMS AND SOLES, SPREADING CENTRIPETALLY TO THE TRUNK AND FACE

PARONYCHIA VS. FELON

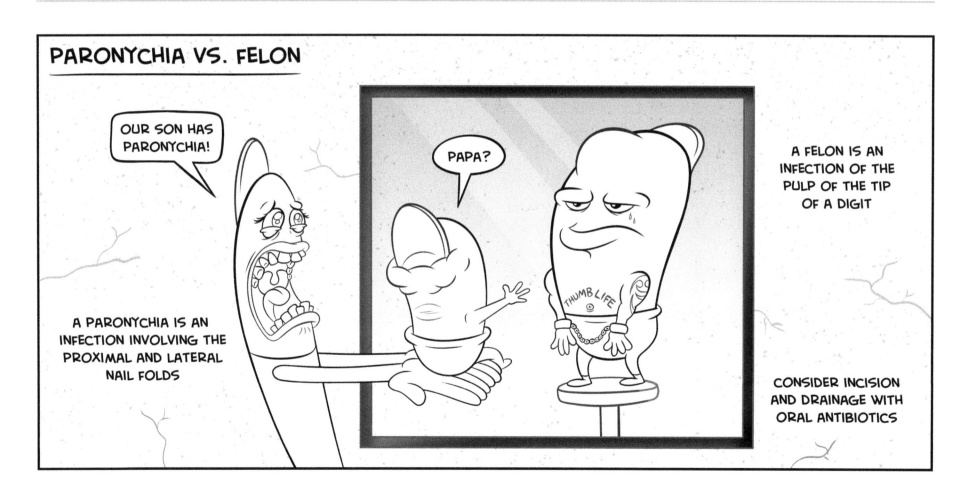

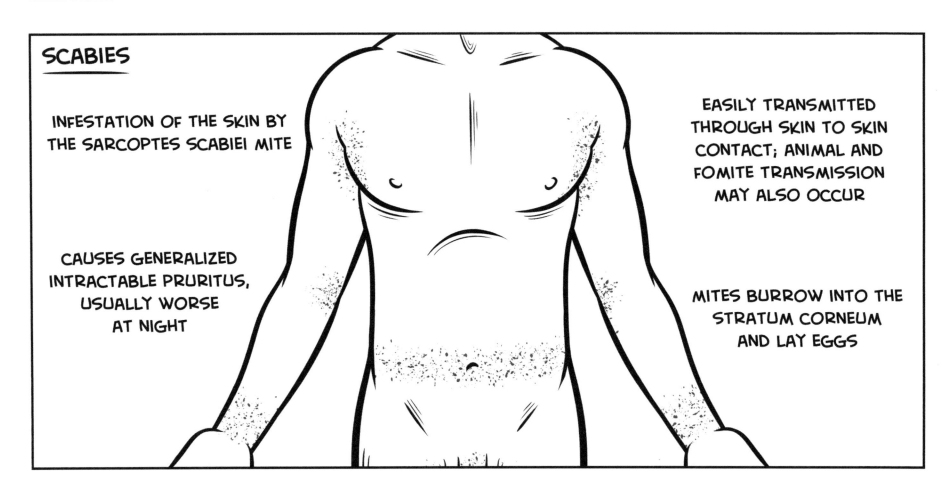

SCABIES

INFESTATION OF THE SKIN BY THE SARCOPTES SCABIEI MITE

EASILY TRANSMITTED THROUGH SKIN TO SKIN CONTACT; ANIMAL AND FOMITE TRANSMISSION MAY ALSO OCCUR

CAUSES GENERALIZED INTRACTABLE PRURITUS, USUALLY WORSE AT NIGHT

MITES BURROW INTO THE STRATUM CORNEUM AND LAY EGGS

SCABIES

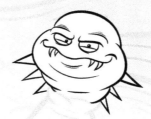

1ST-LINE TREATMENT IS PERMETHRIN 5% APPLIED TO ALL AREAS OF THE BODY FROM THE NECK DOWN AND WASHED OFF AFTER 8-12 HOURS

SYMPTOMS OFTEN PERSIST FOR SEVERAL WEEKS DESPITE EFFECTIVE TREATMENT

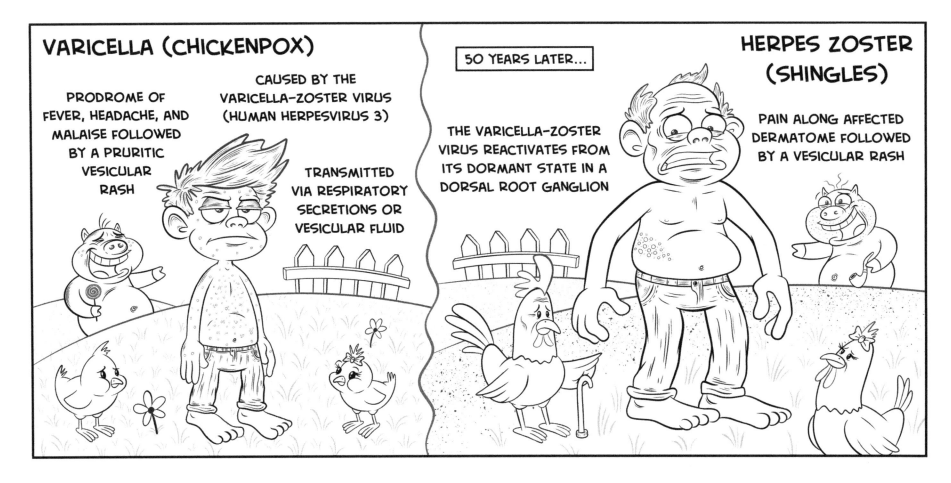

BURNS

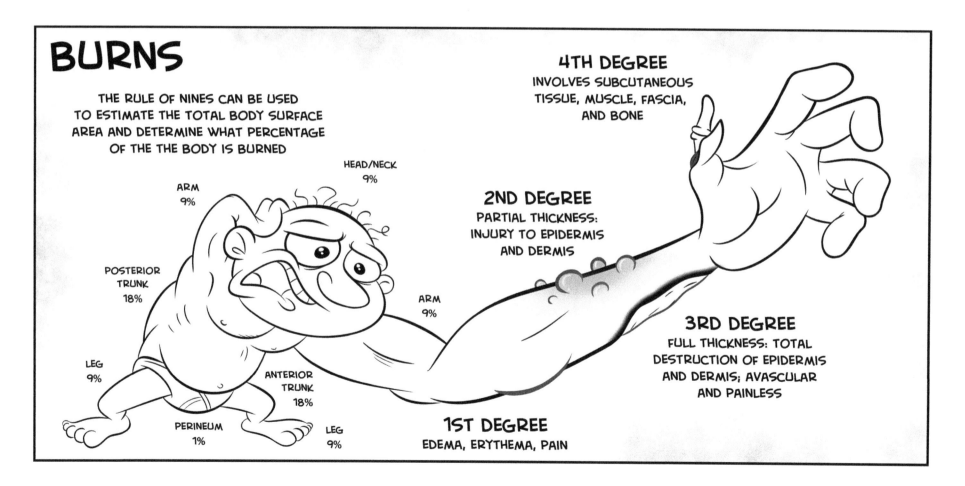

THE RULE OF NINES CAN BE USED TO ESTIMATE THE TOTAL BODY SURFACE AREA AND DETERMINE WHAT PERCENTAGE OF THE THE BODY IS BURNED

HEAD/NECK
9%

ARM
9%

POSTERIOR TRUNK
18%

ARM
9%

LEG
9%

ANTERIOR TRUNK
18%

PERINEUM
1%

LEG
9%

4TH DEGREE
INVOLVES SUBCUTANEOUS TISSUE, MUSCLE, FASCIA, AND BONE

2ND DEGREE
PARTIAL THICKNESS: INJURY TO EPIDERMIS AND DERMIS

3RD DEGREE
FULL THICKNESS: TOTAL DESTRUCTION OF EPIDERMIS AND DERMIS; AVASCULAR AND PAINLESS

1ST DEGREE
EDEMA, ERYTHEMA, PAIN

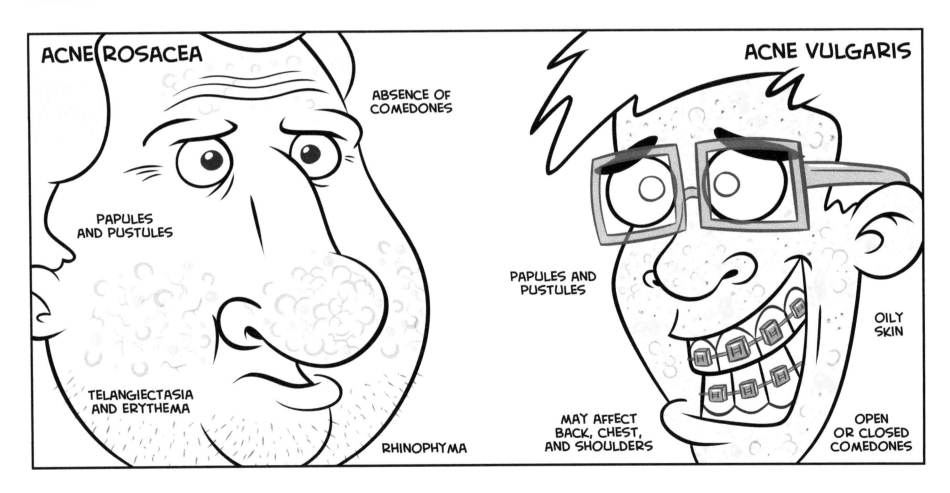

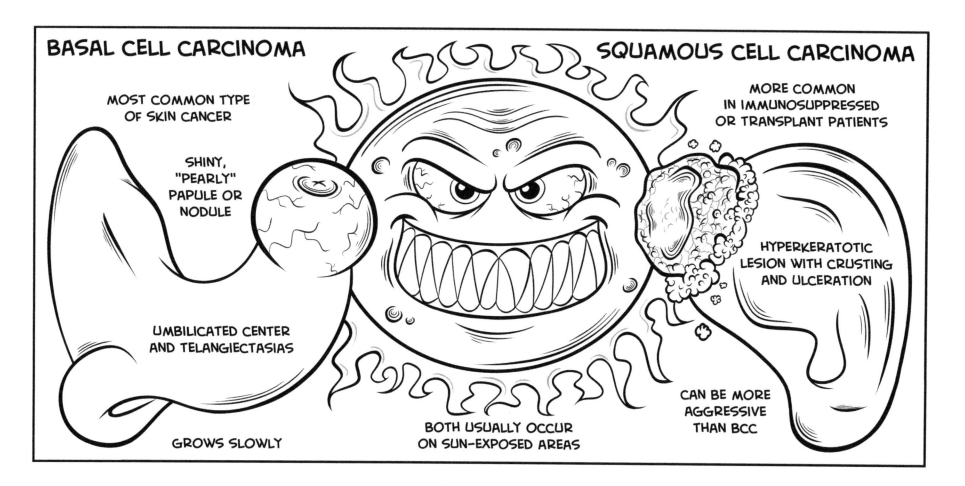

BASAL CELL CARCINOMA

SQUAMOUS CELL CARCINOMA

MOST COMMON TYPE OF SKIN CANCER

SHINY, "PEARLY" PAPULE OR NODULE

UMBILICATED CENTER AND TELANGIECTASIAS

GROWS SLOWLY

MORE COMMON IN IMMUNOSUPPRESSED OR TRANSPLANT PATIENTS

HYPERKERATOTIC LESION WITH CRUSTING AND ULCERATION

CAN BE MORE AGGRESSIVE THAN BCC

BOTH USUALLY OCCUR ON SUN-EXPOSED AREAS

MELANOMA RECOGNITION

UGLY DUCKLING SIGN: A LESION THAT APPEARS TO BE AN OUTLIER IN THE PRESENCE OF SIMILAR-APPEARING MOLES

SIGNS OF MELANOMA (ABCDE RULE):

(A) ASYMMETRY IN SHAPE - ONE HALF UNLIKE THE OTHER

(B) BORDER IRREGULARITY

(C) COLOR VARIABILITY - SHADES OF BROWN, BLACK, GRAY, RED, AND WHITE

(D) DIAMETER GREATER THAN 6 MM

(E) EVOLVING - THE LESION IS CHANGING IN SIZE, SHAPE, OR SHADE OF COLOR

THE FOUR MAJOR TYPES OF MELANOMA ARE SUPERFICIAL SPREADING, NODULAR, LENTIGO MALIGNA, AND ACRAL LENTIGINOUS

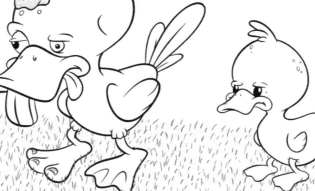

I THINK YOU SHOULD GET THAT CHECKED OUT.

NEUROLOGY AND PSYCHIATRY

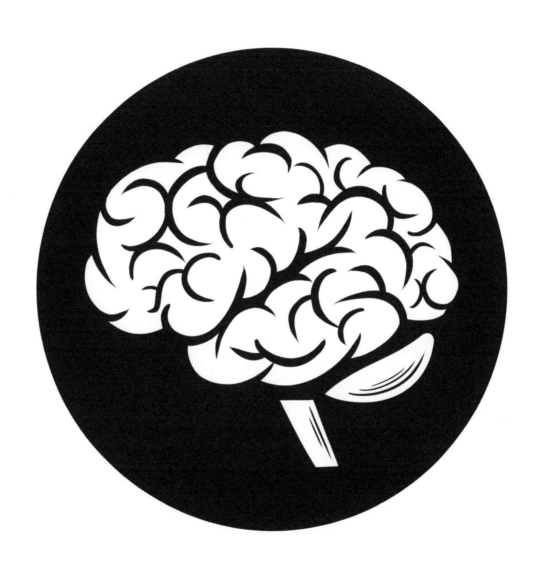

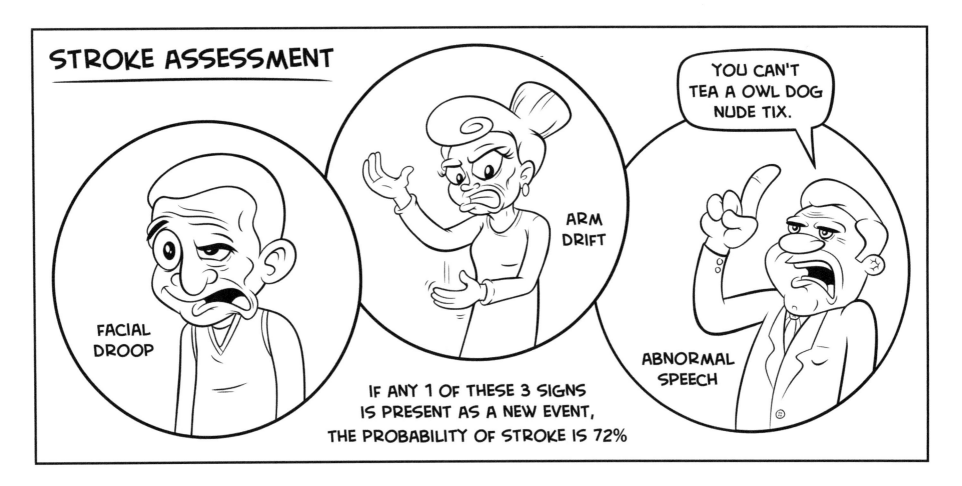

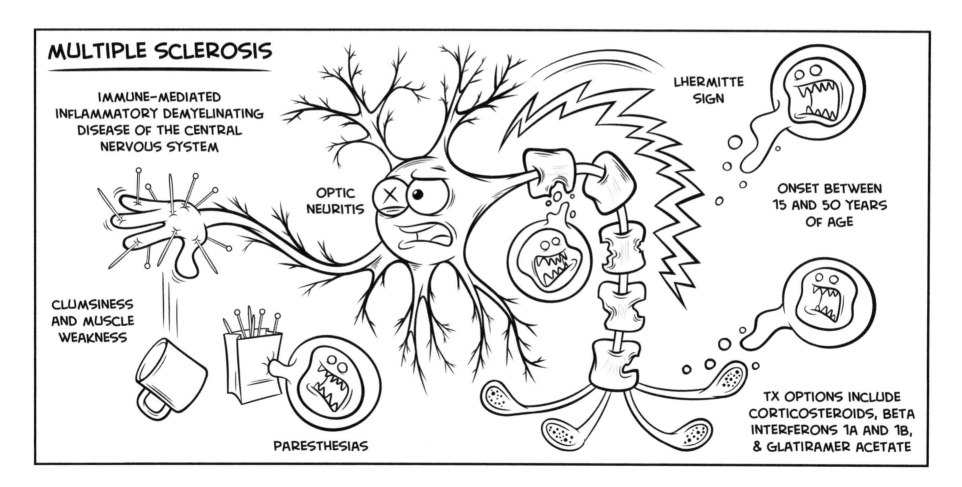

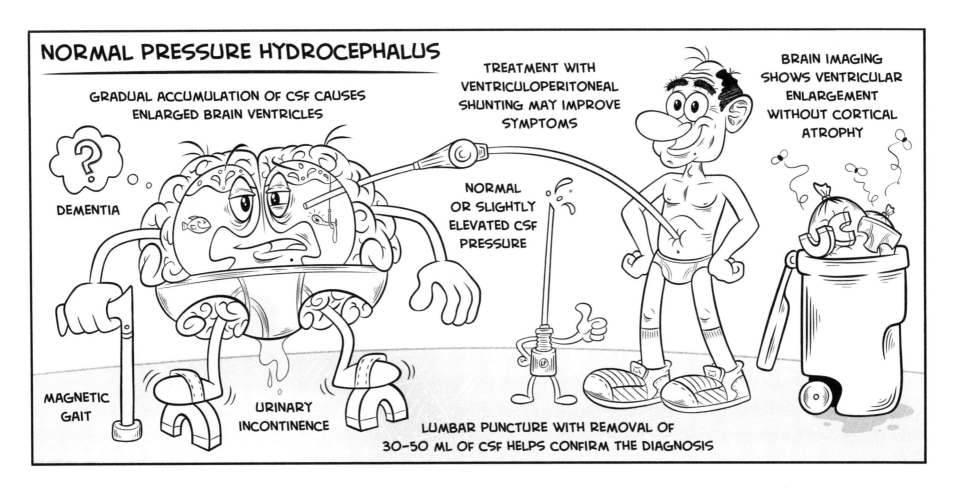

NORMAL PRESSURE HYDROCEPHALUS

GRADUAL ACCUMULATION OF CSF CAUSES
ENLARGED BRAIN VENTRICLES

TREATMENT WITH
VENTRICULOPERITONEAL
SHUNTING MAY IMPROVE
SYMPTOMS

BRAIN IMAGING
SHOWS VENTRICULAR
ENLARGEMENT
WITHOUT CORTICAL
ATROPHY

DEMENTIA

NORMAL
OR SLIGHTLY
ELEVATED CSF
PRESSURE

MAGNETIC
GAIT

URINARY
INCONTINENCE

LUMBAR PUNCTURE WITH REMOVAL OF
30-50 ML OF CSF HELPS CONFIRM THE DIAGNOSIS

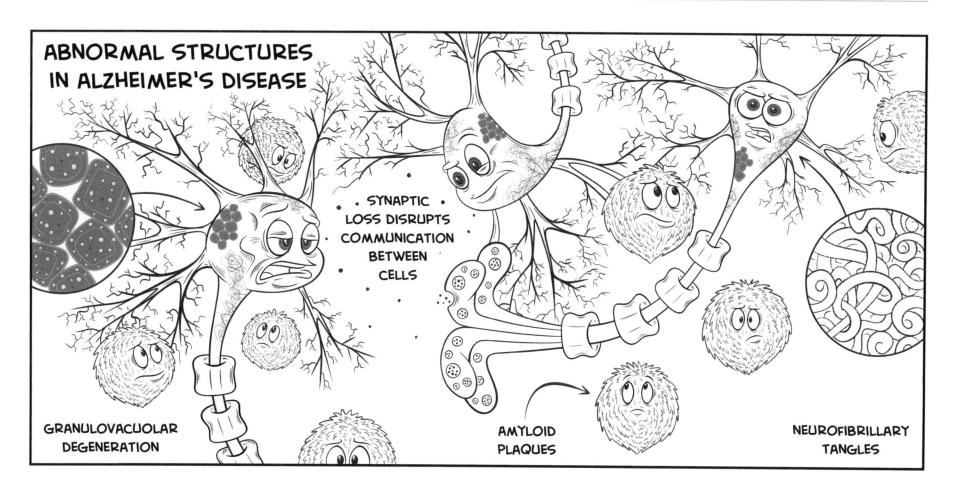

GRADING DEEP TENDON REFLEXES

0: ABSENT REFLEX

1: HYPOACTIVE

2: NORMAL

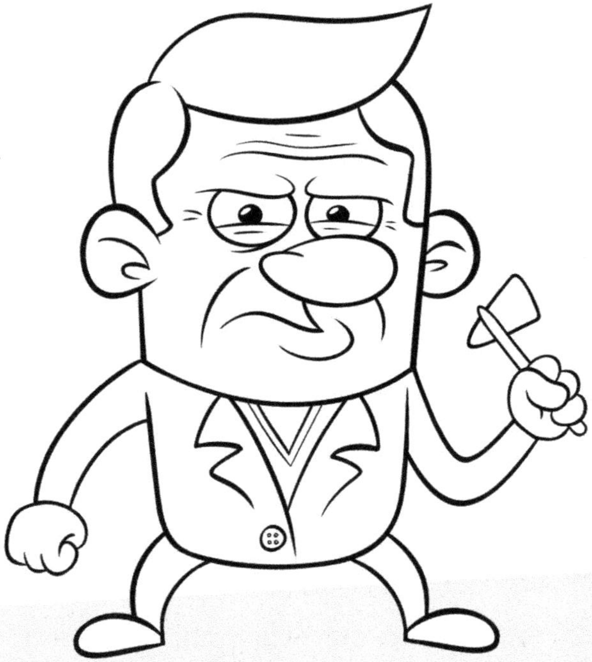

3: HYPERACTIVE

4: NONSUSTAINED CLONUS

5: SUSTAINED CLONUS

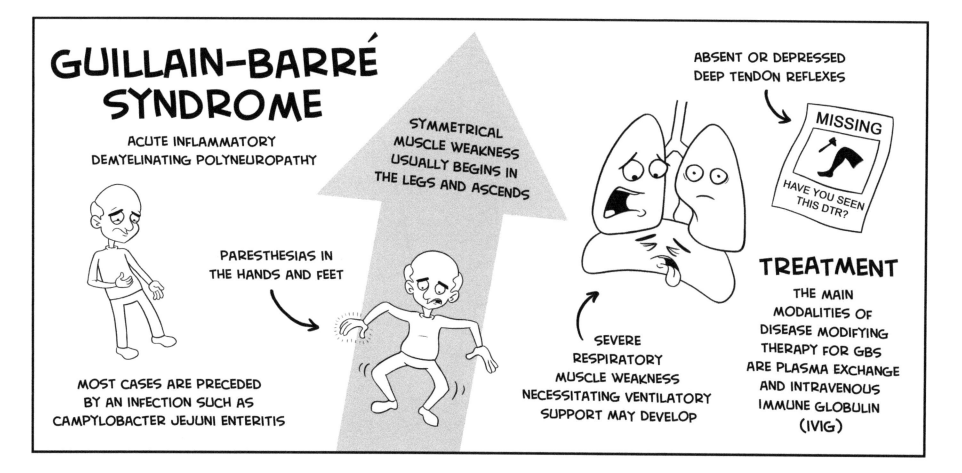

GUILLAIN-BARRÉ SYNDROME

ACUTE INFLAMMATORY DEMYELINATING POLYNEUROPATHY

MOST CASES ARE PRECEDED BY AN INFECTION SUCH AS CAMPYLOBACTER JEJUNI ENTERITIS

PARESTHESIAS IN THE HANDS AND FEET

SYMMETRICAL MUSCLE WEAKNESS USUALLY BEGINS IN THE LEGS AND ASCENDS

SEVERE RESPIRATORY MUSCLE WEAKNESS NECESSITATING VENTILATORY SUPPORT MAY DEVELOP

ABSENT OR DEPRESSED DEEP TENDON REFLEXES

MISSING

HAVE YOU SEEN THIS DTR?

TREATMENT

THE MAIN MODALITIES OF DISEASE MODIFYING THERAPY FOR GBS ARE PLASMA EXCHANGE AND INTRAVENOUS IMMUNE GLOBULIN (IVIG)

CRANIAL NERVES

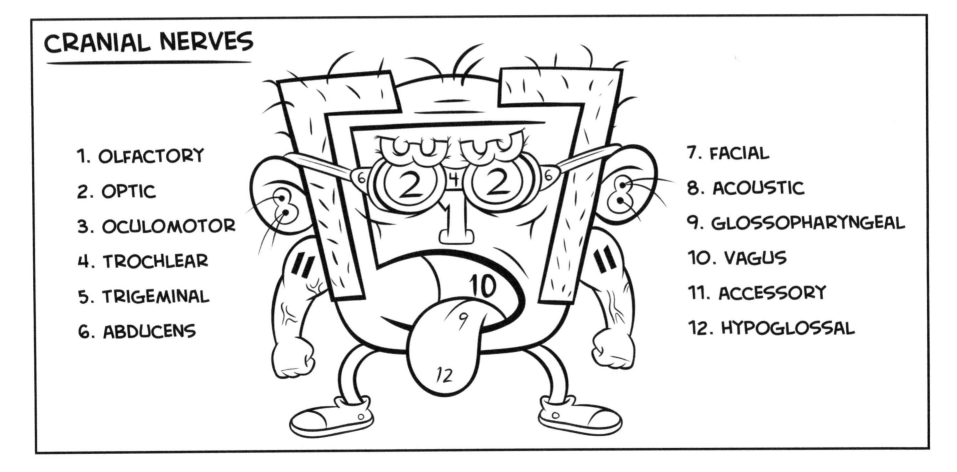

1. OLFACTORY
2. OPTIC
3. OCULOMOTOR
4. TROCHLEAR
5. TRIGEMINAL
6. ABDUCENS

7. FACIAL
8. ACOUSTIC
9. GLOSSOPHARYNGEAL
10. VAGUS
11. ACCESSORY
12. HYPOGLOSSAL

CRANIAL NERVES

1. The olfactory nerve (CN I) contains special sensory neurons concerned with smell.

2. The optic nerve (CN II) contains sensory neurons dedicated to vision.

3. The oculomotor nerve (CN III) provides motor function for all eye muscles except those supplied by cranial nerves IV and VI.

4. The trochlear nerve (CN IV) provides motor function to the superior oblique muscle of the eye.

5. The trigeminal nerve (CN V) is the principal sensory supply to the head (face, teeth, sinuses, etc.); it also provides motor function to the muscles of mastication.

6. The abducens nerve (CN VI) provides motor function to the lateral rectus muscle of the eye.

7. The facial nerve (CN VII) provides motor innervation to the muscles of facial expression, lacrimal gland, submaxillary gland, sublingual gland, as well as sensory supply to the anterior two-thirds of the tongue.

8. The acoustic nerve (CN VIII), also known as the vestibulocochlear nerve, provides sensory innervation for hearing and equilibrium.

9. The glossopharyngeal nerve (CN IX) provides motor innervation to the pharyngeal musculature and sensory function to the posterior one-third of the tongue and pharynx.

10. The vagus nerve (CN X) provides motor innervation to the heart, lungs, and gastrointestinal tract. It also provides sensory innervation to the heart, respiratory tract, gastrointestinal tract, and external ear.

11. The accessory nerve (CN XI) provides motor function to the sternocleidomastoid and trapezius muscles.

12. The hypoglossal nerve (CN XII) is a pure motor nerve that innervates the muscles of the tongue.

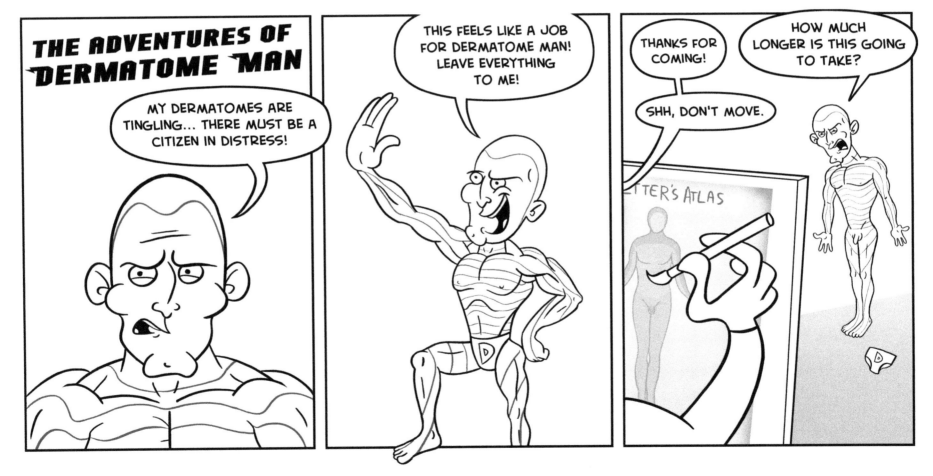

DERMATOMES

NERVE ROOT

PERIPHERAL NERVE

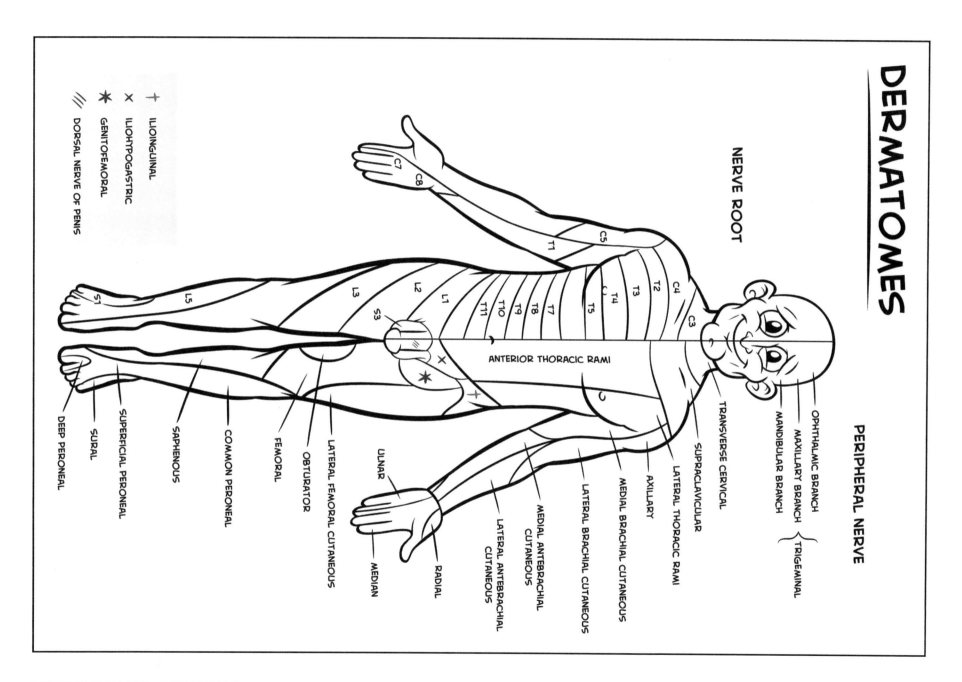

/// DORSAL NERVE OF PENIS
✱ GENITOFEMORAL
✕ ILIOHYPOGASTRIC
✝ ILIOINGUINAL

C7
C8
C5
T1
C4
T2
T3
C
T4
T5
C3
L2
L3
L1
T11
T10
T9
T8
T7
S3
S1
L5

ANTERIOR THORACIC RAMI

OPHTHALMIC BRANCH
MAXILLARY BRANCH ⎤ TRIGEMINAL
MANDIBULAR BRANCH ⎦
TRANSVERSE CERVICAL
SUPRACLAVICULAR
LATERAL THORACIC RAMI
AXILLARY
MEDIAL BRACHIAL CUTANEOUS
LATERAL BRACHIAL CUTANEOUS
MEDIAL ANTEBRACHIAL CUTANEOUS
LATERAL ANTEBRACHIAL CUTANEOUS
RADIAL
MEDIAN
ULNAR

DEEP PERONEAL
SURAL
SUPERFICIAL PERONEAL
SAPHENOUS
COMMON PERONEAL
FEMORAL
OBTURATOR
LATERAL FEMORAL CUTANEOUS

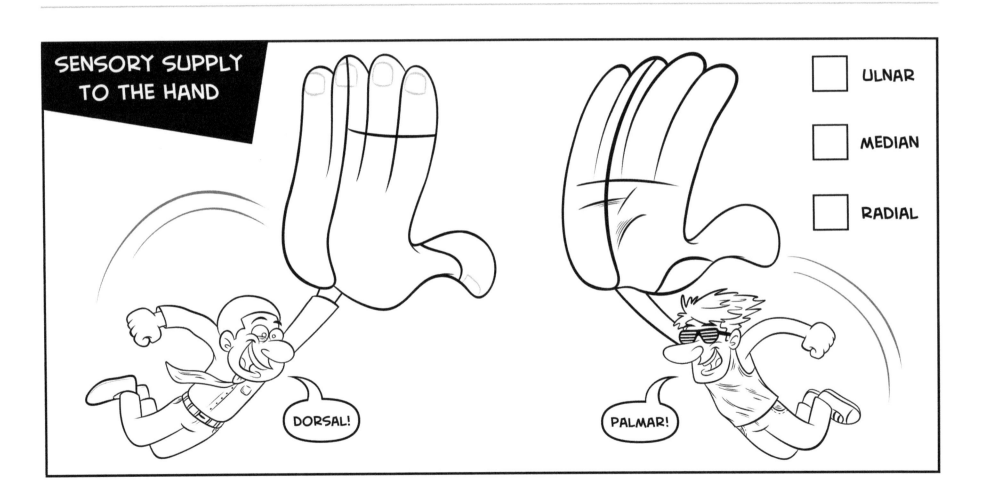

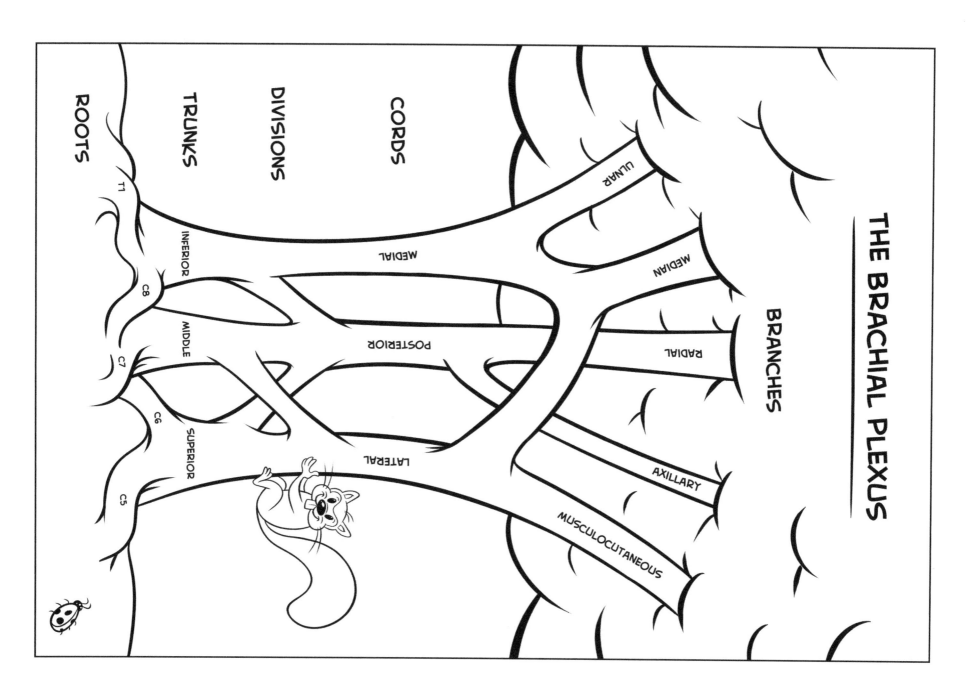

THE BRACHIAL PLEXUS

ROOTS

TRUNKS

DIVISIONS

CORDS

BRANCHES

T1

C8

C7

C6

C5

INFERIOR

MIDDLE

SUPERIOR

MEDIAL

POSTERIOR

LATERAL

ULNAR

MEDIAN

RADIAL

AXILLARY

MUSCULOCUTANEOUS

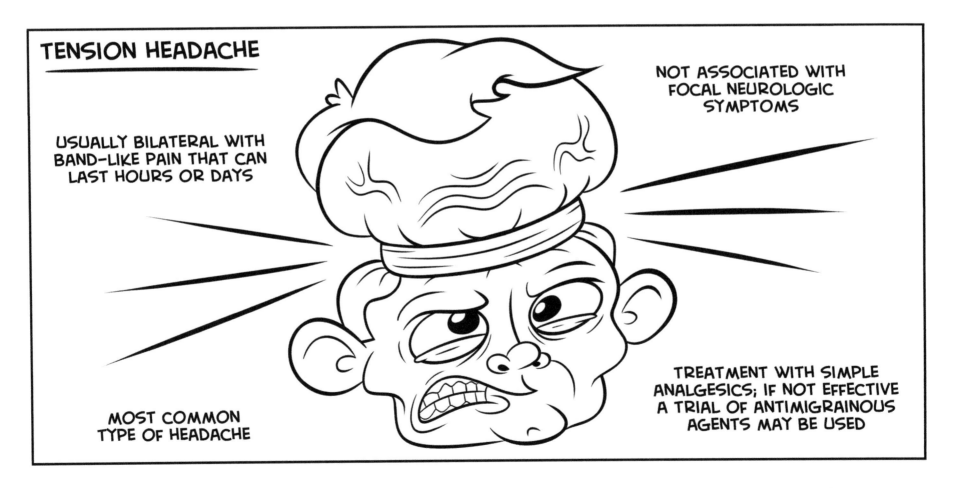

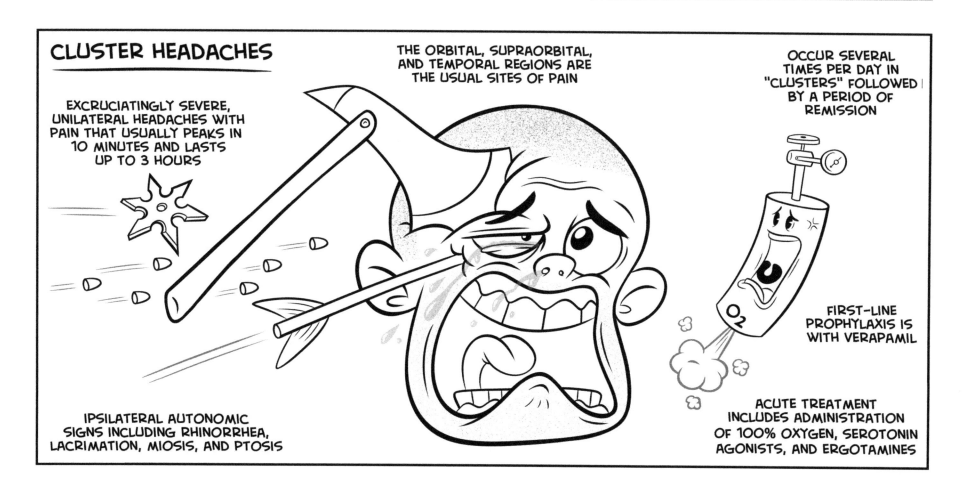

CLUSTER HEADACHES

EXCRUCIATINGLY SEVERE, UNILATERAL HEADACHES WITH PAIN THAT USUALLY PEAKS IN 10 MINUTES AND LASTS UP TO 3 HOURS

THE ORBITAL, SUPRAORBITAL, AND TEMPORAL REGIONS ARE THE USUAL SITES OF PAIN

OCCUR SEVERAL TIMES PER DAY IN "CLUSTERS" FOLLOWED BY A PERIOD OF REMISSION

IPSILATERAL AUTONOMIC SIGNS INCLUDING RHINORRHEA, LACRIMATION, MIOSIS, AND PTOSIS

FIRST-LINE PROPHYLAXIS IS WITH VERAPAMIL

ACUTE TREATMENT INCLUDES ADMINISTRATION OF 100% OXYGEN, SEROTONIN AGONISTS, AND ERGOTAMINES

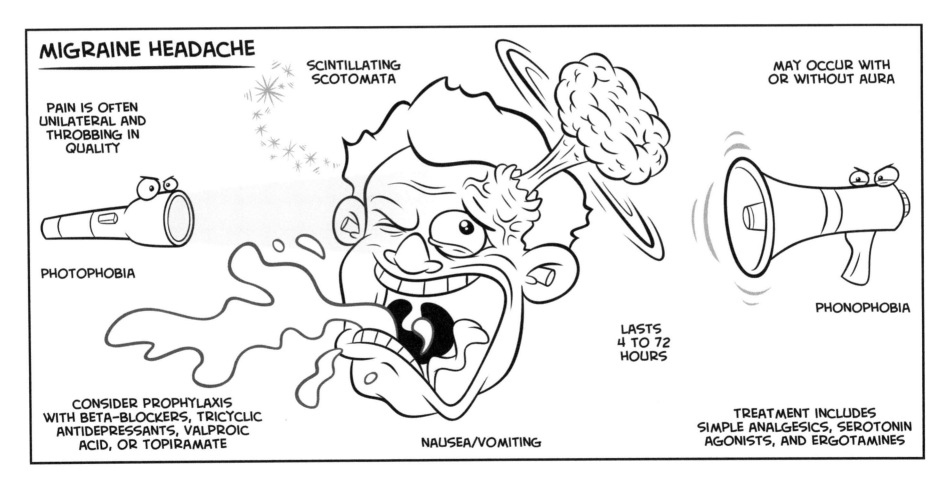

MIGRAINE HEADACHE

SCINTILLATING SCOTOMATA

MAY OCCUR WITH OR WITHOUT AURA

PAIN IS OFTEN UNILATERAL AND THROBBING IN QUALITY

PHOTOPHOBIA

PHONOPHOBIA

LASTS 4 TO 72 HOURS

CONSIDER PROPHYLAXIS WITH BETA-BLOCKERS, TRICYCLIC ANTIDEPRESSANTS, VALPROIC ACID, OR TOPIRAMATE

NAUSEA/VOMITING

TREATMENT INCLUDES SIMPLE ANALGESICS, SEROTONIN AGONISTS, AND ERGOTAMINES

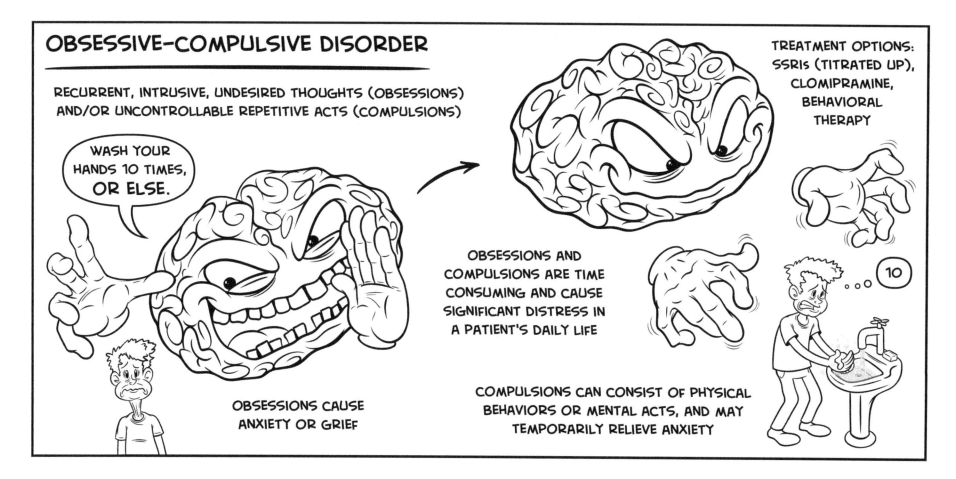

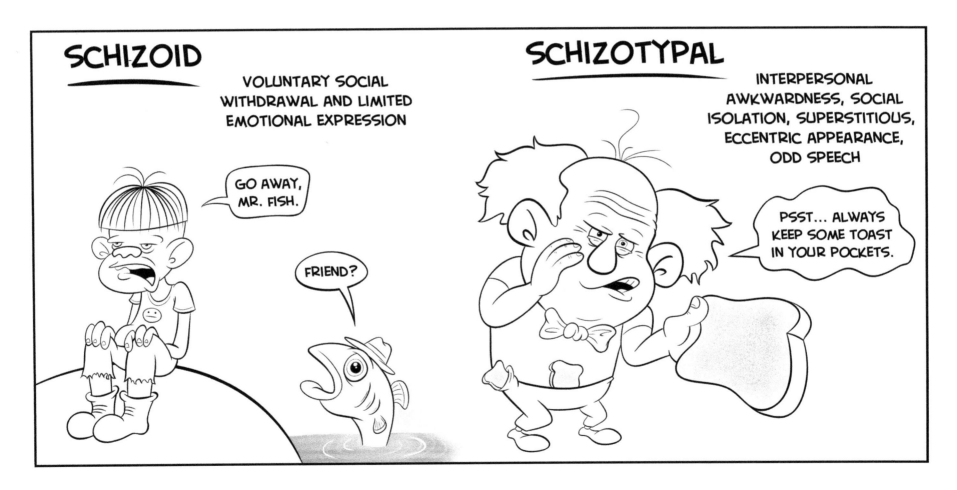

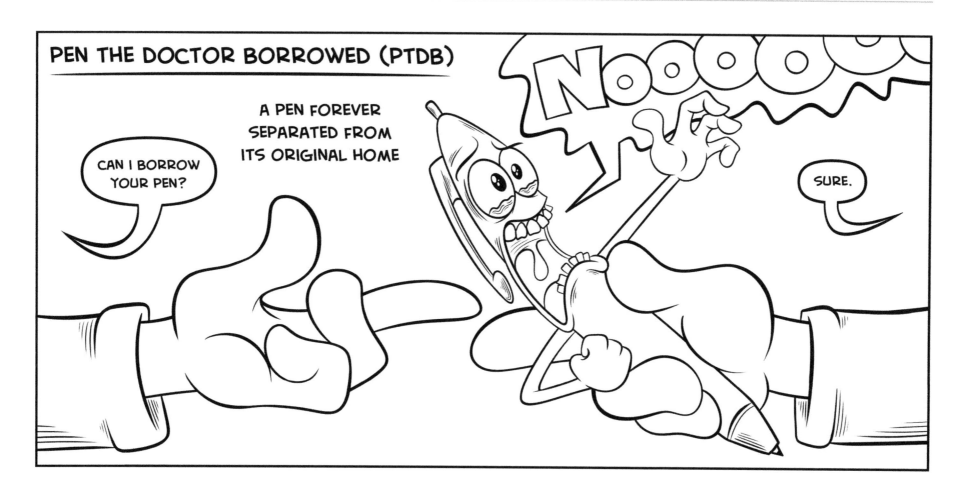

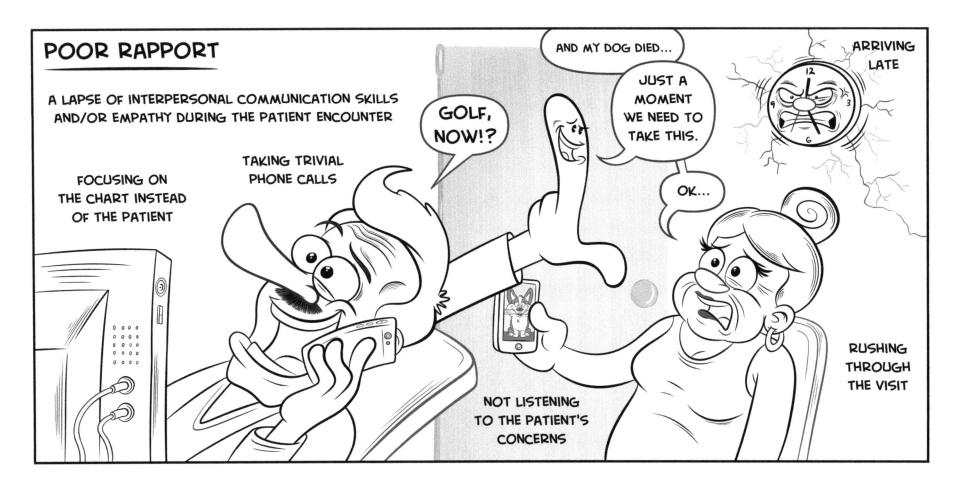

HEMATOLOGY AND ONCOLOGY

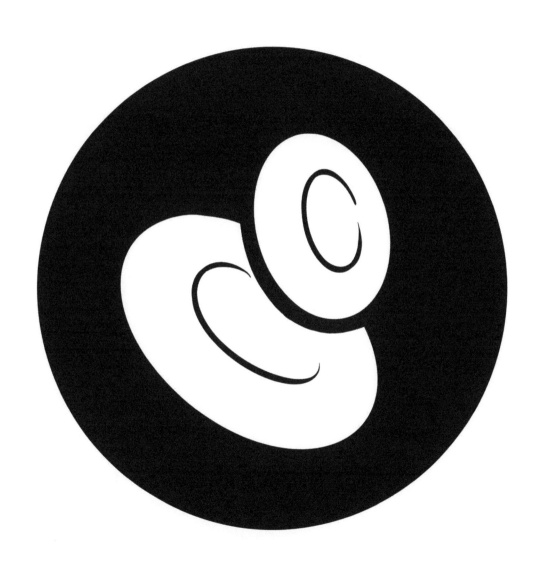

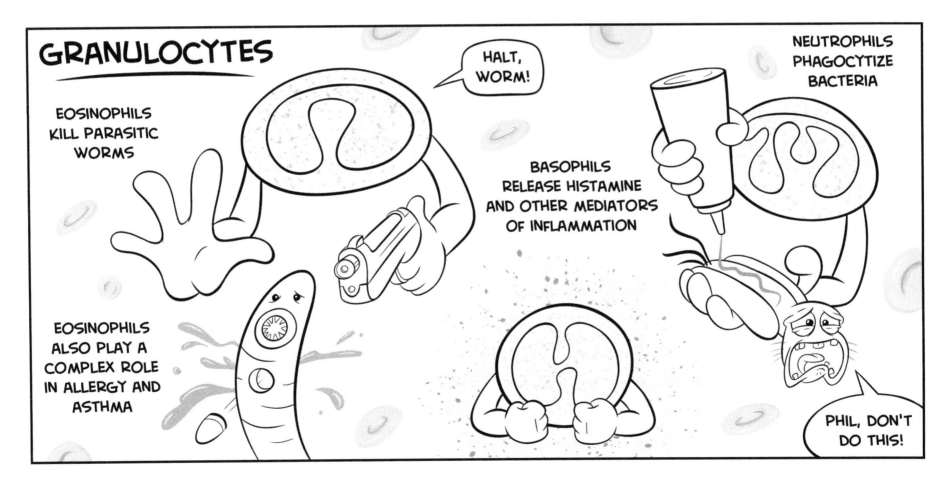

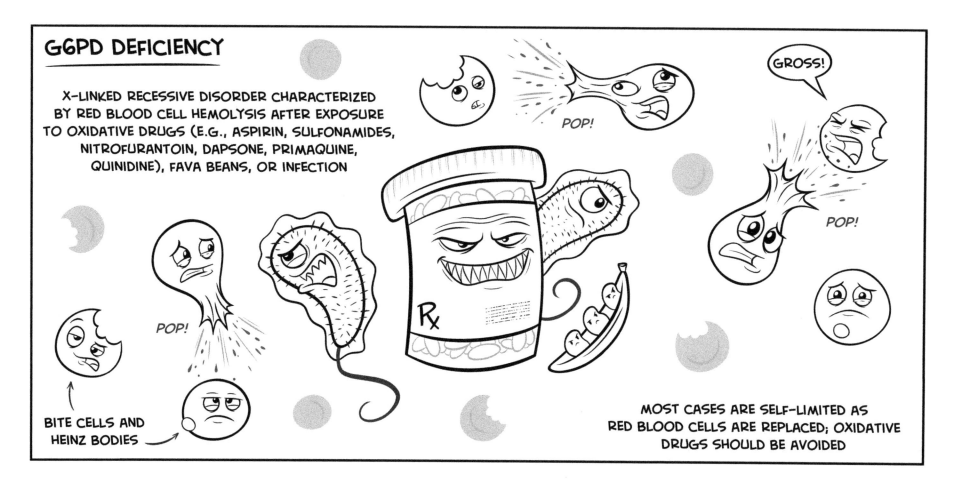

G6PD DEFICIENCY

X-LINKED RECESSIVE DISORDER CHARACTERIZED BY RED BLOOD CELL HEMOLYSIS AFTER EXPOSURE TO OXIDATIVE DRUGS (E.G., ASPIRIN, SULFONAMIDES, NITROFURANTOIN, DAPSONE, PRIMAQUINE, QUINIDINE), FAVA BEANS, OR INFECTION

BITE CELLS AND HEINZ BODIES

MOST CASES ARE SELF-LIMITED AS RED BLOOD CELLS ARE REPLACED; OXIDATIVE DRUGS SHOULD BE AVOIDED

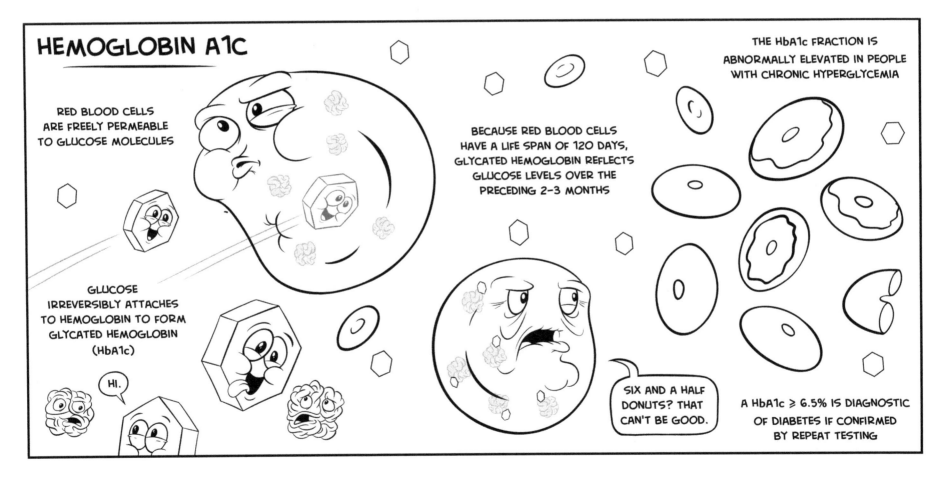

VON WILLEBRAND DISEASE

MOST COMMON INHERITED BLEEDING DISORDER

PATIENTS MAY PRESENT WITH MUCOCUTANEOUS BLEEDING (E.G., EPISTAXIS, EASY BRUISING, MENORRHAGIA, GI BLEEDING)

VON WILLEBRAND FACTOR (VWF) ACTS AS A CARRIER PROTEIN FOR FACTOR VIII IN PLASMA

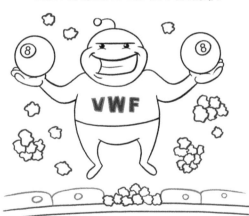

VWF ALSO HELPS WITH PLATELET AGGREGATION AND ADHESION TO DAMAGED ENDOTHELIUM

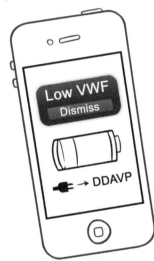

TYPE 1: DEFICIENCY OF VWF (MOST COMMON TYPE)

TREATMENT: DESMOPRESSIN OR CRYOPRECIPITATE

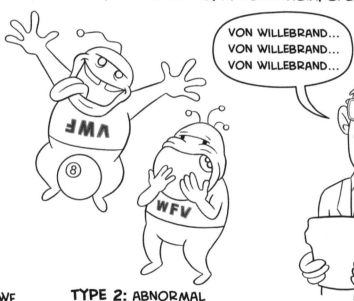

TYPE 2: ABNORMAL AND DYSFUNCTIONAL VWF

TYPE 3: VWF IS ABSENT

TREATMENT: FACTOR VIII CONCENTRATE OR CRYOPRECIPITATE

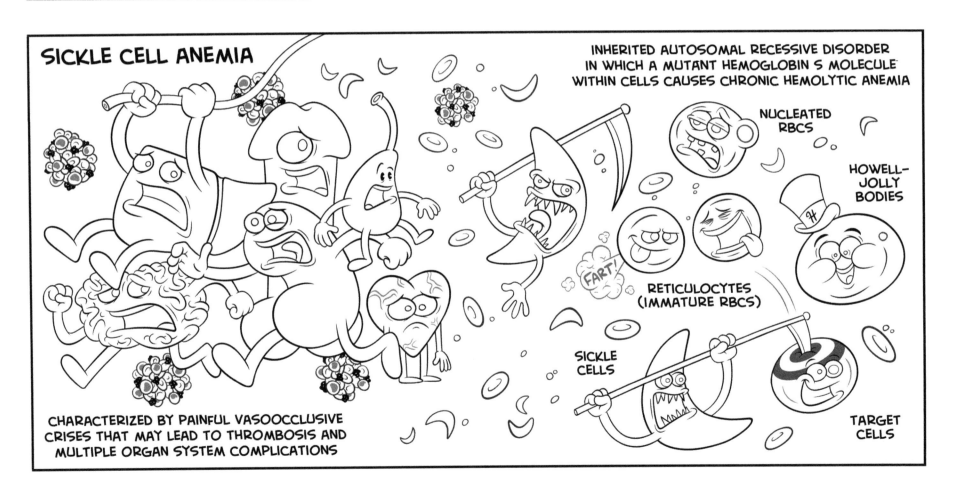

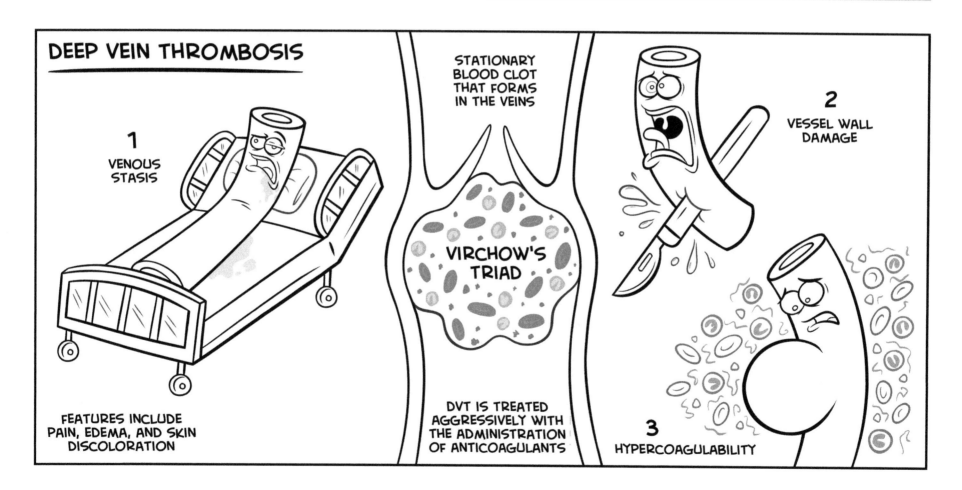

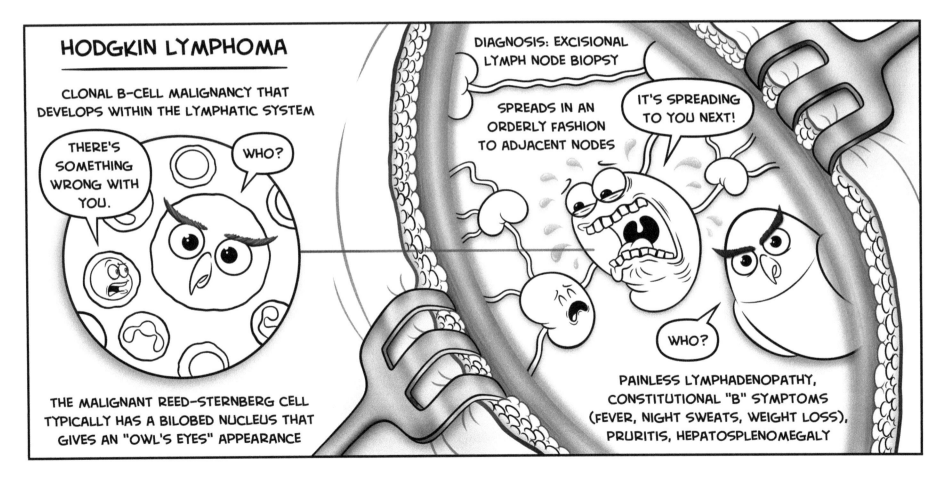

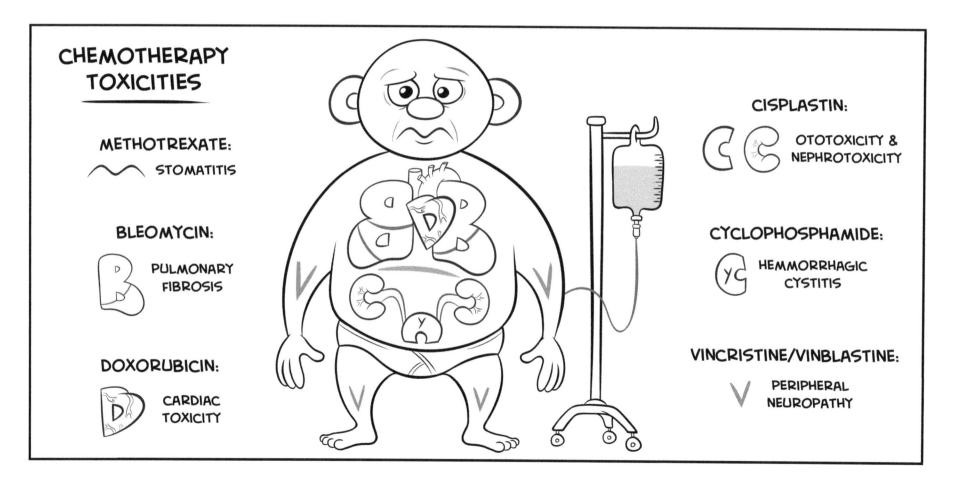

CHEMOTHERAPY TOXICITIES

METHOTREXATE: STOMATITIS

BLEOMYCIN: PULMONARY FIBROSIS

DOXORUBICIN: CARDIAC TOXICITY

CISPLASTIN: OTOTOXICITY & NEPHROTOXICITY

CYCLOPHOSPHAMIDE: HEMMORRHAGIC CYSTITIS

VINCRISTINE/VINBLASTINE: PERIPHERAL NEUROPATHY

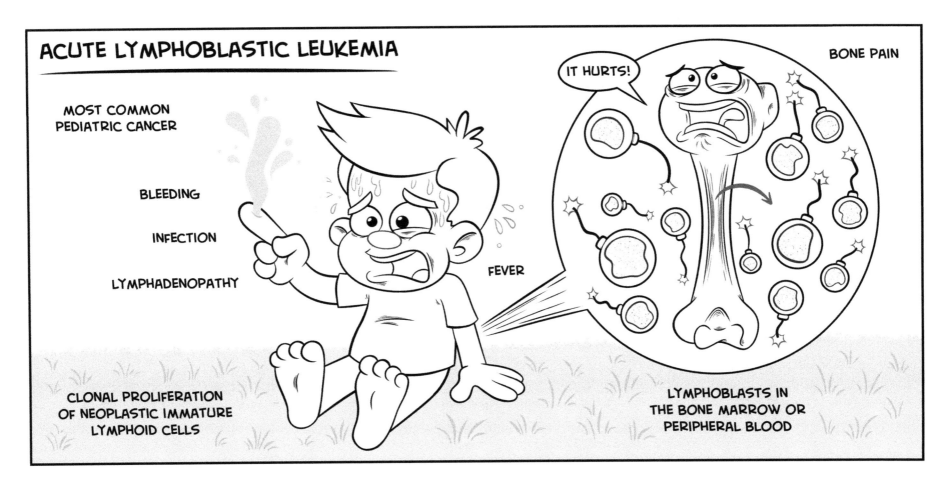

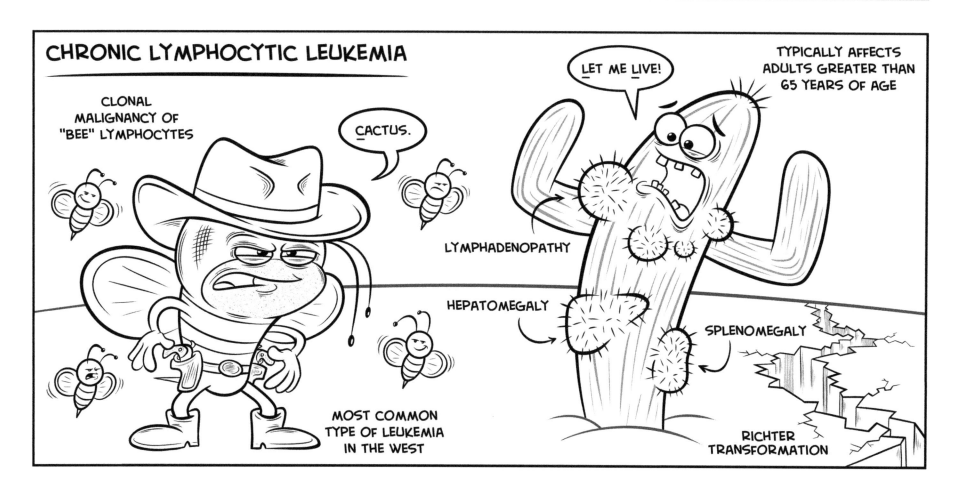

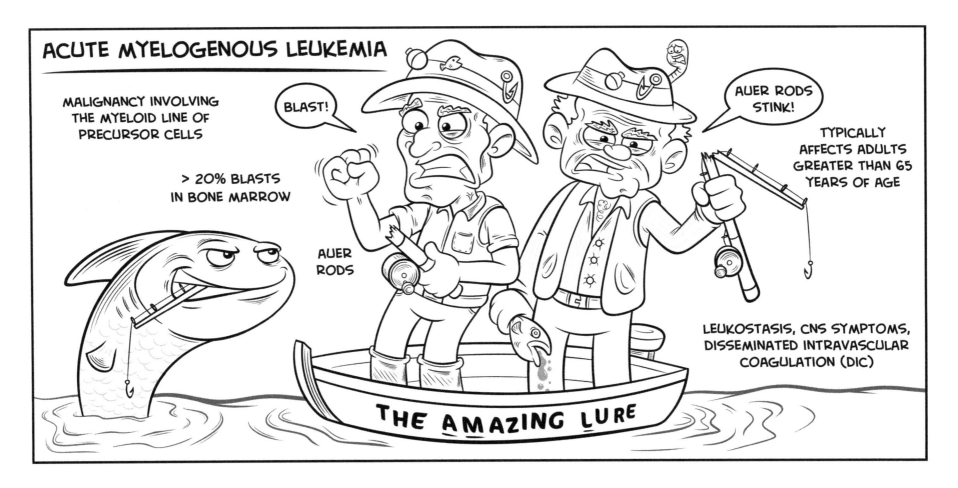

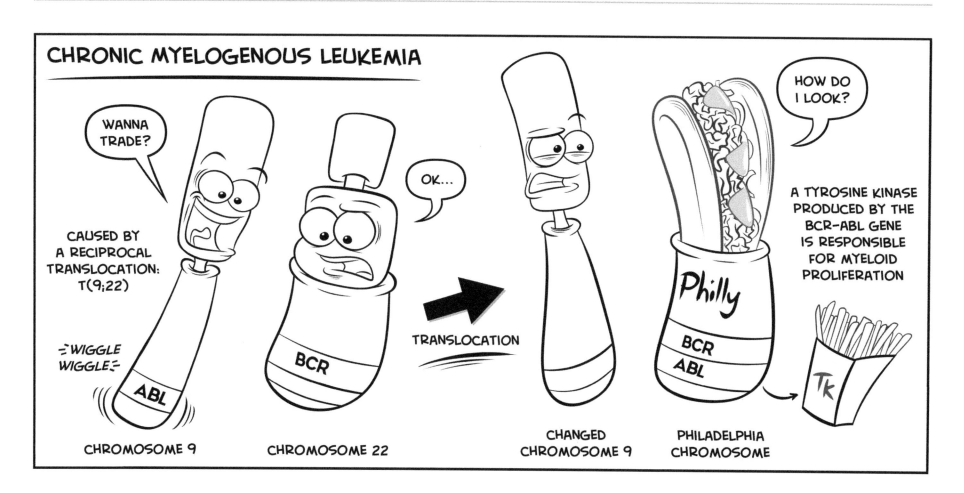

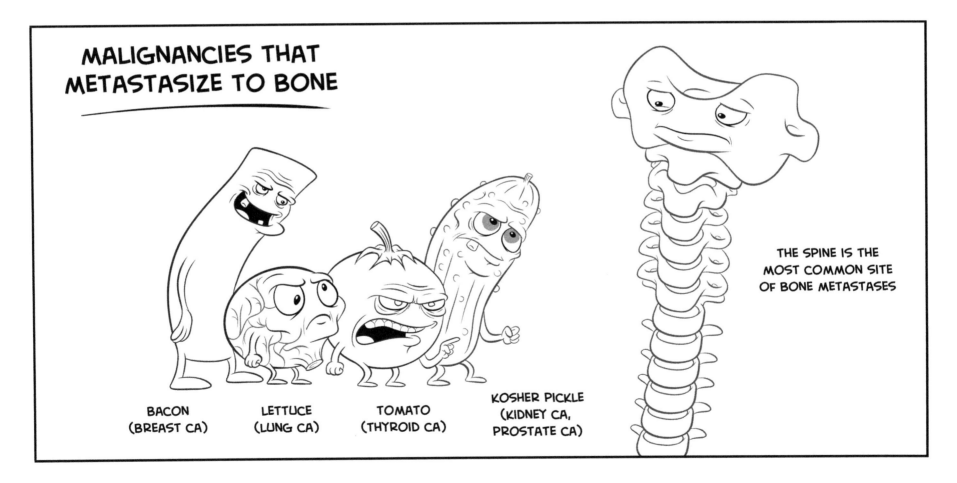

ORTHOPEDICS

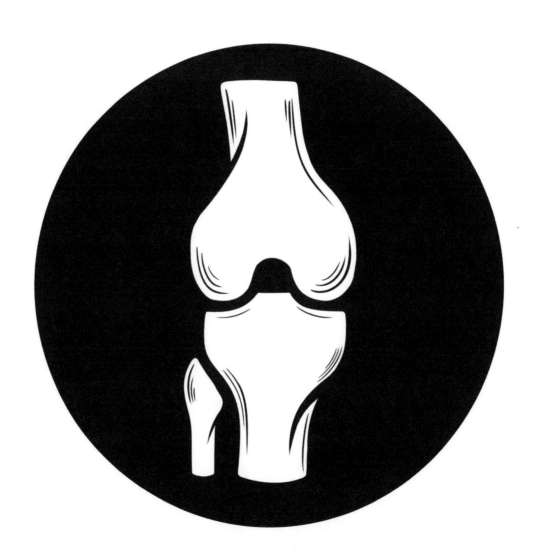

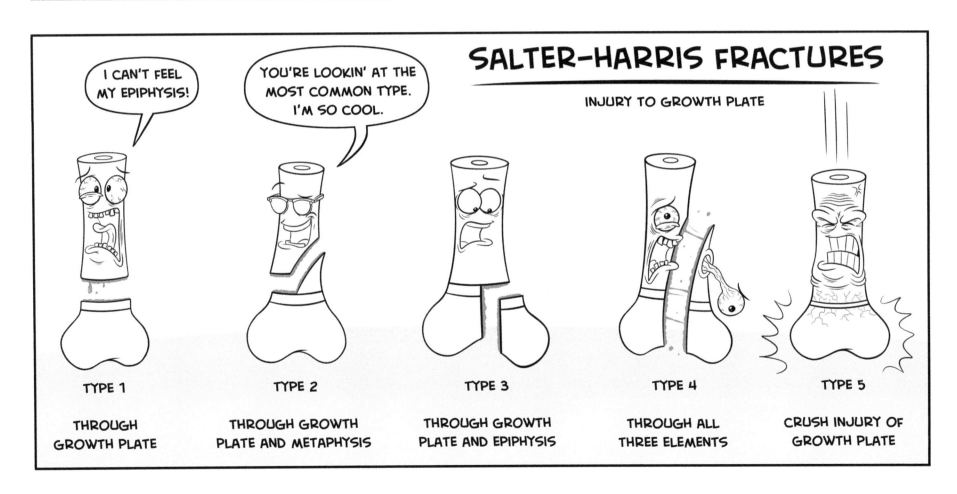

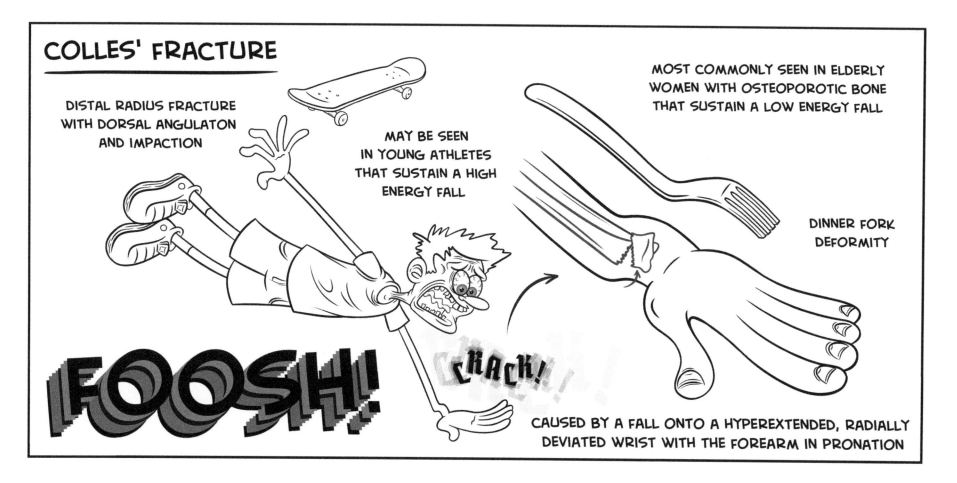

COLLES' FRACTURE

DISTAL RADIUS FRACTURE WITH DORSAL ANGULATON AND IMPACTION

MAY BE SEEN IN YOUNG ATHLETES THAT SUSTAIN A HIGH ENERGY FALL

MOST COMMONLY SEEN IN ELDERLY WOMEN WITH OSTEOPOROTIC BONE THAT SUSTAIN A LOW ENERGY FALL

DINNER FORK DEFORMITY

FOOSH!

CRACK!

CAUSED BY A FALL ONTO A HYPEREXTENDED, RADIALLY DEVIATED WRIST WITH THE FOREARM IN PRONATION

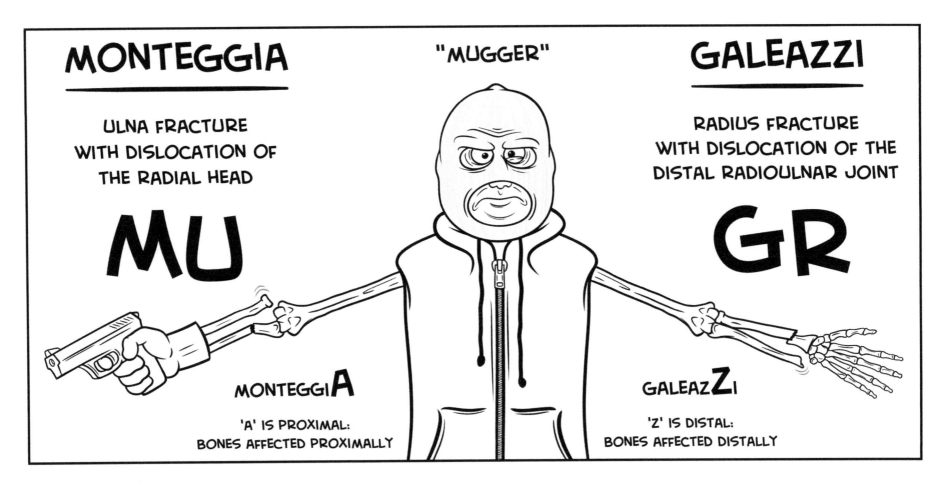

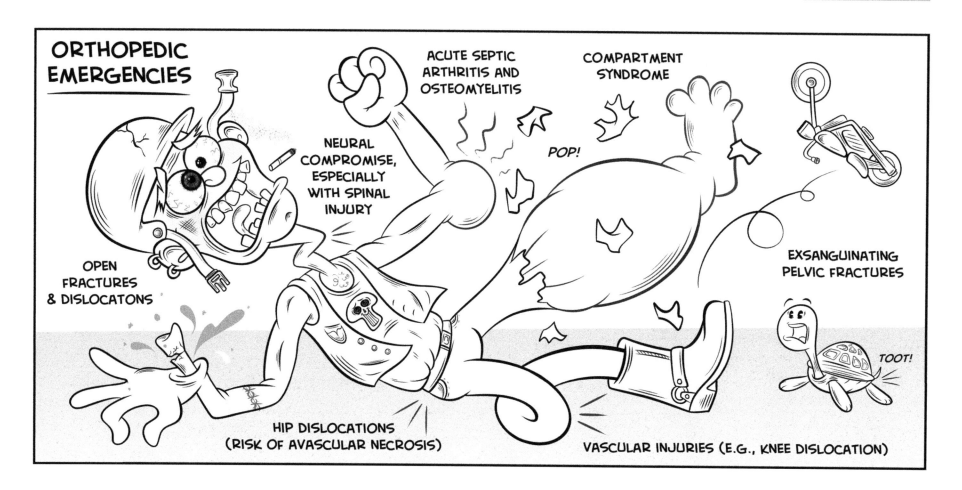

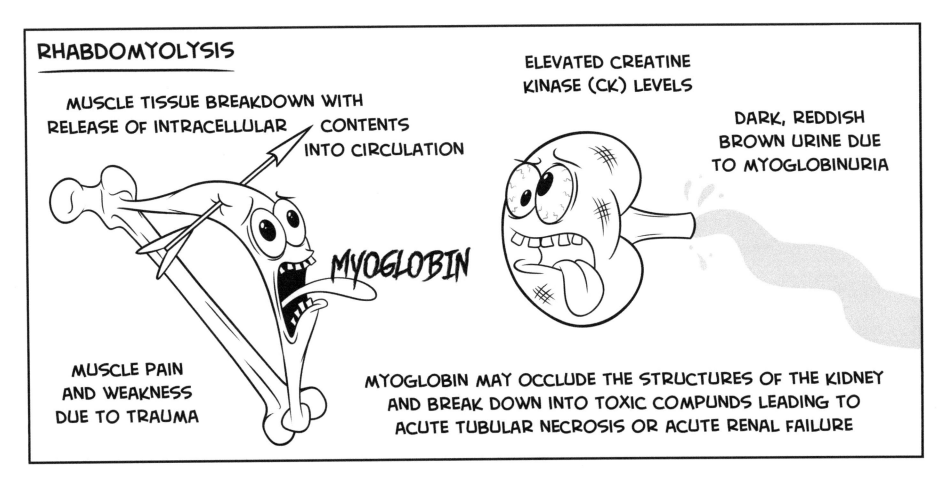

RHABDOMYOLYSIS

MUSCLE TISSUE BREAKDOWN WITH RELEASE OF INTRACELLULAR CONTENTS INTO CIRCULATION

MUSCLE PAIN AND WEAKNESS DUE TO TRAUMA

MYOGLOBIN

ELEVATED CREATINE KINASE (CK) LEVELS

DARK, REDDISH BROWN URINE DUE TO MYOGLOBINURIA

MYOGLOBIN MAY OCCLUDE THE STRUCTURES OF THE KIDNEY AND BREAK DOWN INTO TOXIC COMPUNDS LEADING TO ACUTE TUBULAR NECROSIS OR ACUTE RENAL FAILURE

THE FEMUR

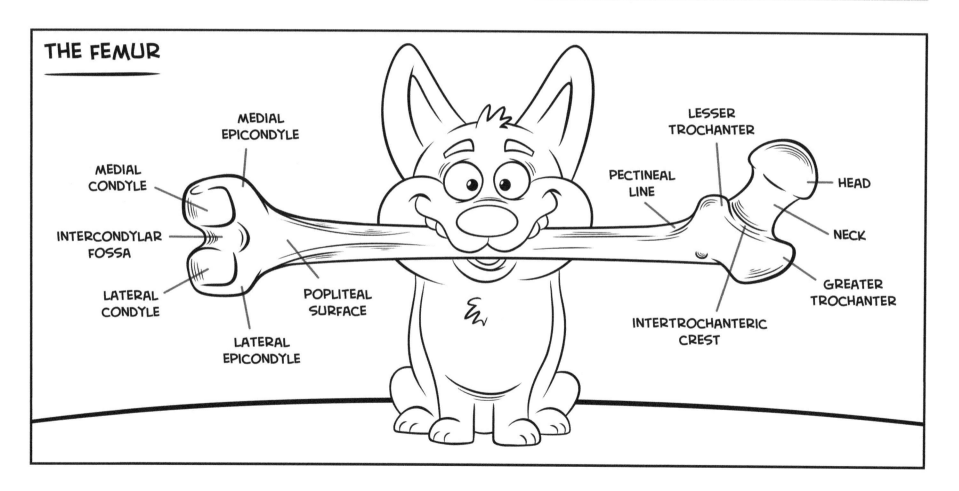

MEDIAL CONDYLE

MEDIAL EPICONDYLE

INTERCONDYLAR FOSSA

LATERAL CONDYLE

POPLITEAL SURFACE

LATERAL EPICONDYLE

LESSER TROCHANTER

PECTINEAL LINE

HEAD

NECK

GREATER TROCHANTER

INTERTROCHANTERIC CREST

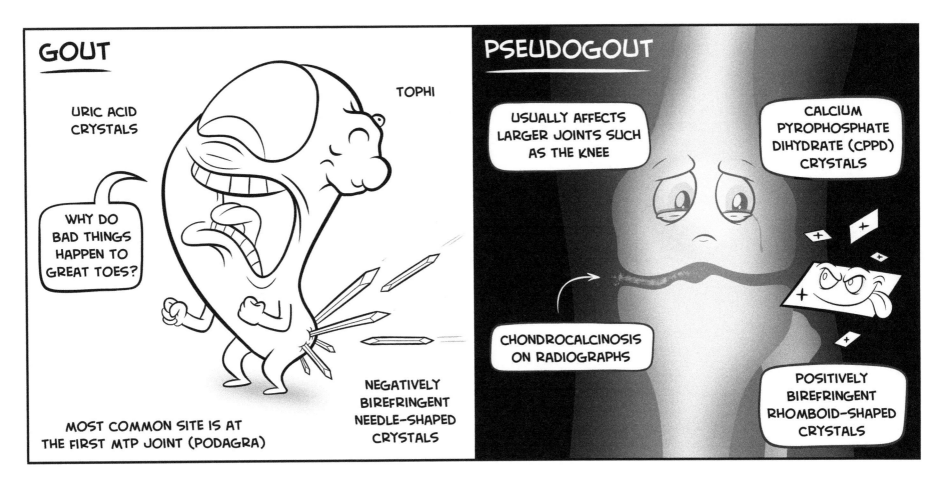

PAIN RELIEF

NSAIDS

IBUPROFEN
(ADVIL, MOTRIN)
NAPROXEN
(ALEVE)

TYLENOL
WITH CODEINE

(TYLENOL 3)

TRAMADOL

(ULTRAM): WEAK
OPIOID AGONIST

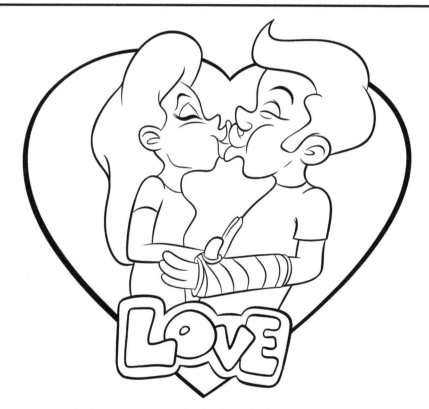

ACTIVATION OF THE NUCLEUS ACCUMBENS

HYDROCODONE

MILD OPIOID
AGONIST AVAILABLE IN
TABLETS CONTAINING
ACETAMINOPHEN:
(NORCO, VICODIN,
LORTAB)

OXYCODONE

MODERATE OPIOID
AGONIST AVAILABLE
IN TABLETS CONTAINING
ACETAMINOPHEN:
(PERCOCET)

HYDROMORPHONE

(DILAUDID): STRONG
OPIOID AGONIST

KNEE ALIGNMENT

LATER IN LIFE, CARTILAGE LOSS DUE TO OSTEOARTHRITIS USUALLY BEGINS IN THE MEDIAL ASPECT OF THE TIBIOFEMORAL JOINT. AS A RESULT, VARUS ANGULATION OCCURS MORE COMMONLY THAN VALGUS

PHYSIOLOGIC GENU VALGUM (KNOCK-KNEES) IS PART OF NORMAL DEVELOPMENT BETWEEN TWO AND FIVE YEARS OF AGE AND ALSO RESOLVES SPONTANEOUSLY

PHYSIOLOGIC GENU VARUM (BOWLEGS) GENERALLY RESOLVES SPONTANEOUSLY

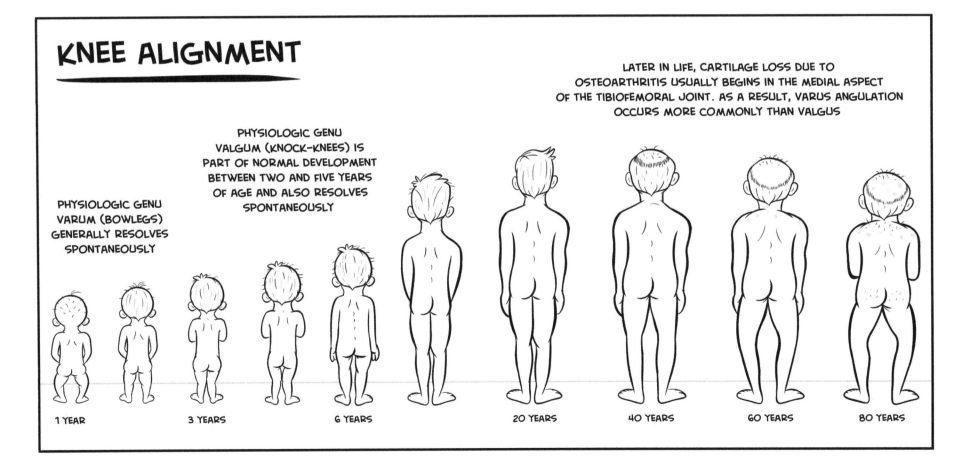

1 YEAR   3 YEARS   6 YEARS   20 YEARS   40 YEARS   60 YEARS   80 YEARS

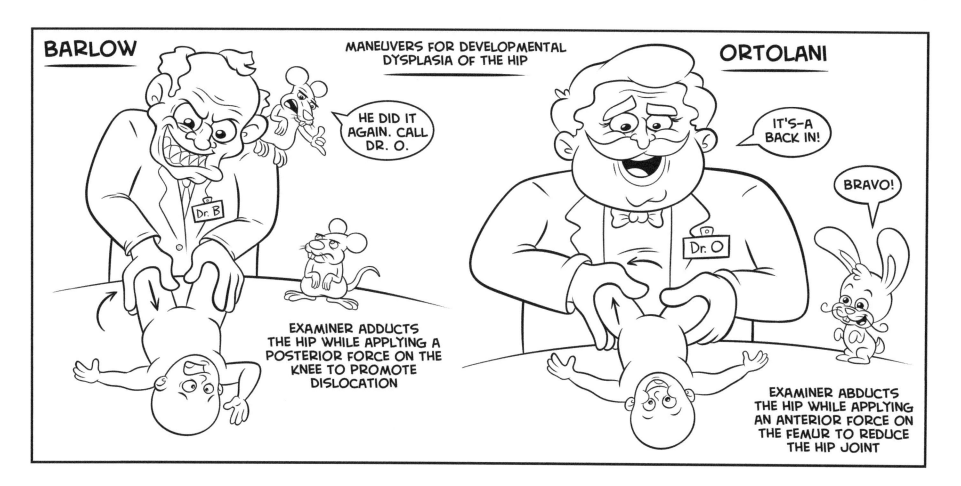

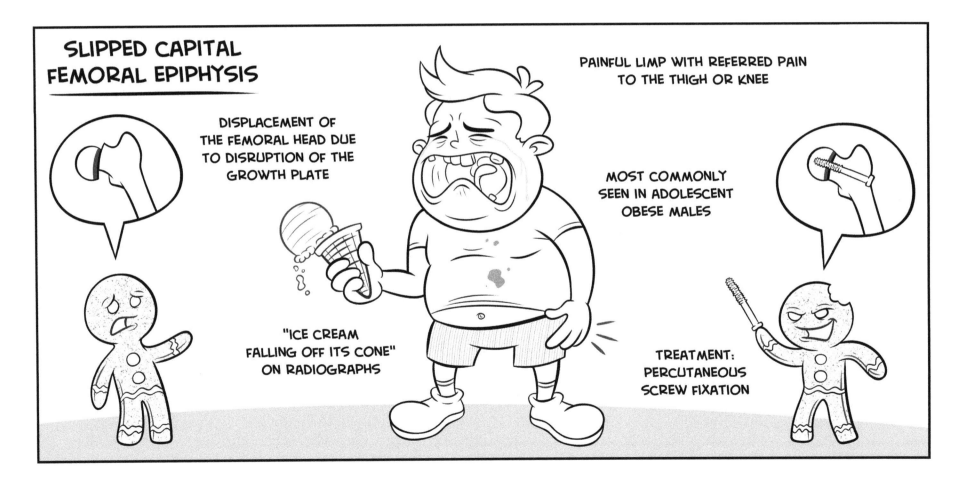

SCOLIOSIS

A COBB ANGLE OF 10 DEGREES OR MORE DEFINES SCOLIOSIS

LATERAL CURVATURE OF THE SPINE

MODERATE CURVES (20 TO 40 DEGREES) ARE TREATED WITH PT AND BRACING

COBB ANGLE →

SEVERE CURVES GREATER THAN 40 DEGREES MAY REQUIRE SURGERY

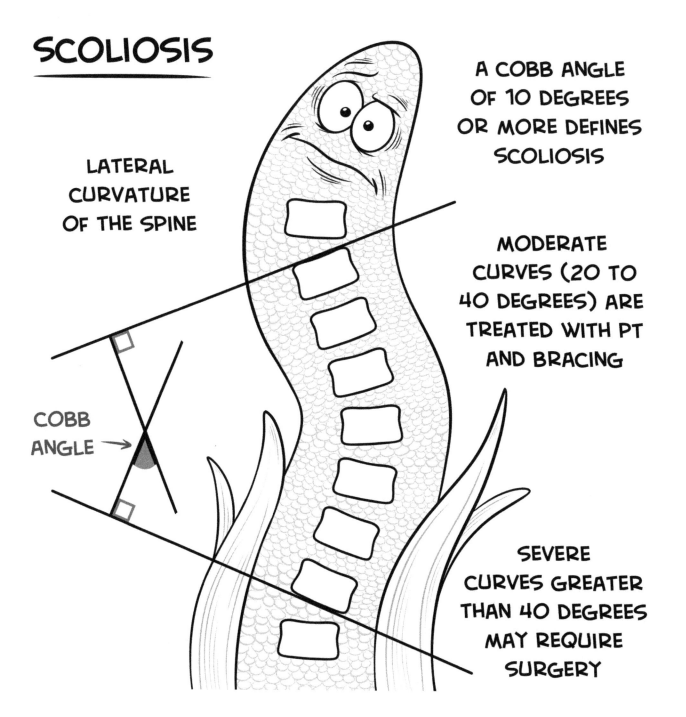

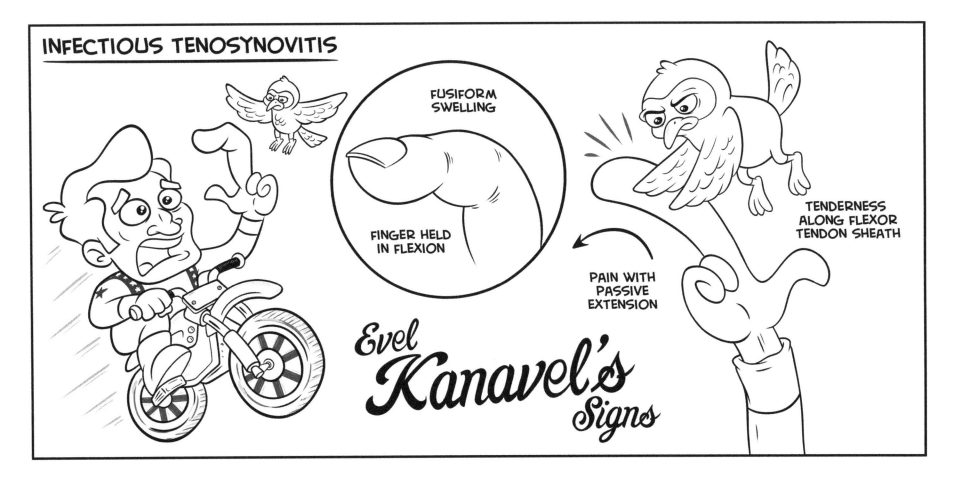

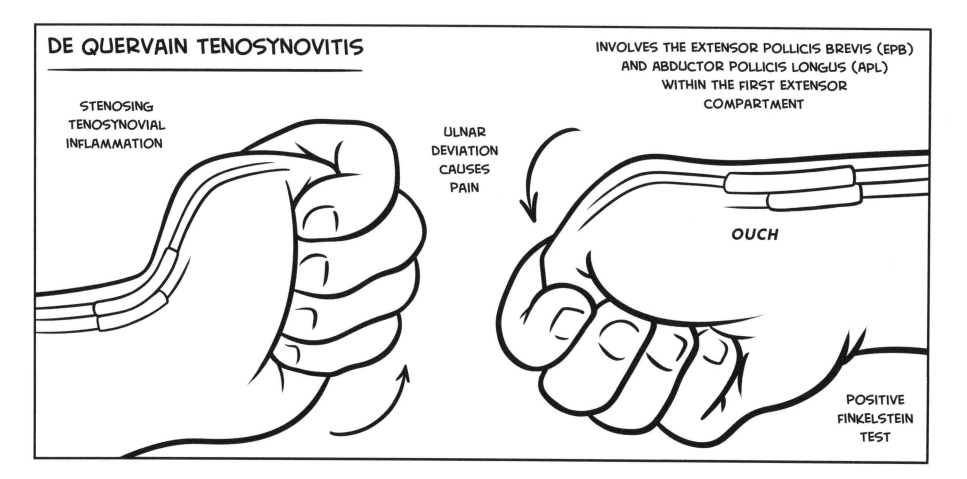

DE QUERVAIN TENOSYNOVITIS

INVOLVES THE EXTENSOR POLLICIS BREVIS (EPB)
AND ABDUCTOR POLLICIS LONGUS (APL)
WITHIN THE FIRST EXTENSOR
COMPARTMENT

STENOSING
TENOSYNOVIAL
INFLAMMATION

ULNAR
DEVIATION
CAUSES
PAIN

OUCH

POSITIVE
FINKELSTEIN
TEST

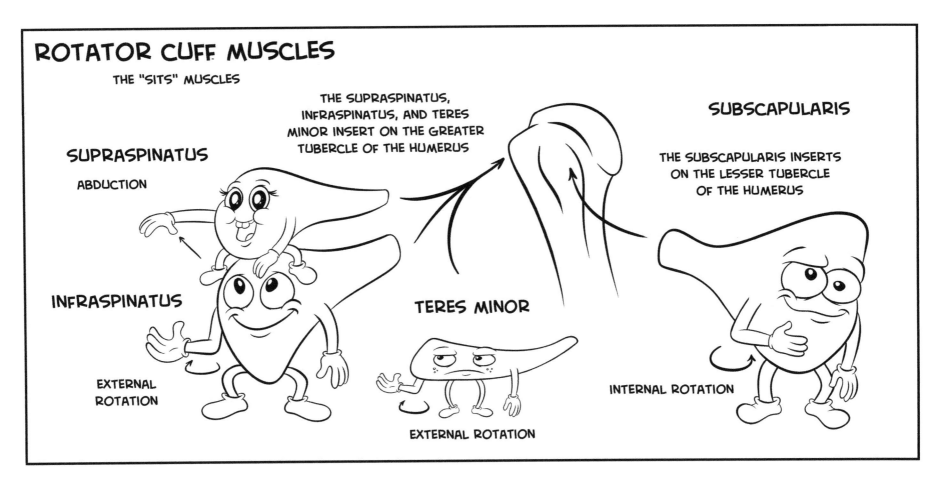

ROTATOR CUFF MUSCLES

THE "SITS" MUSCLES

THE SUPRASPINATUS, INFRASPINATUS, AND TERES MINOR INSERT ON THE GREATER TUBERCLE OF THE HUMERUS

SUBSCAPULARIS

THE SUBSCAPULARIS INSERTS ON THE LESSER TUBERCLE OF THE HUMERUS

SUPRASPINATUS

ABDUCTION

INFRASPINATUS

EXTERNAL ROTATION

TERES MINOR

EXTERNAL ROTATION

INTERNAL ROTATION

RHEUMATOLOGY

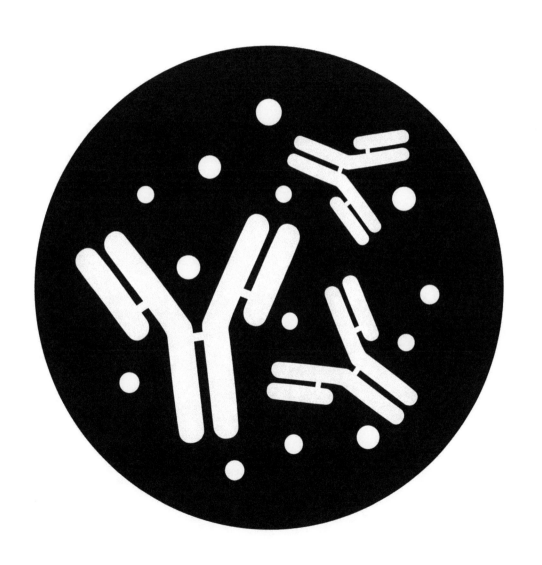

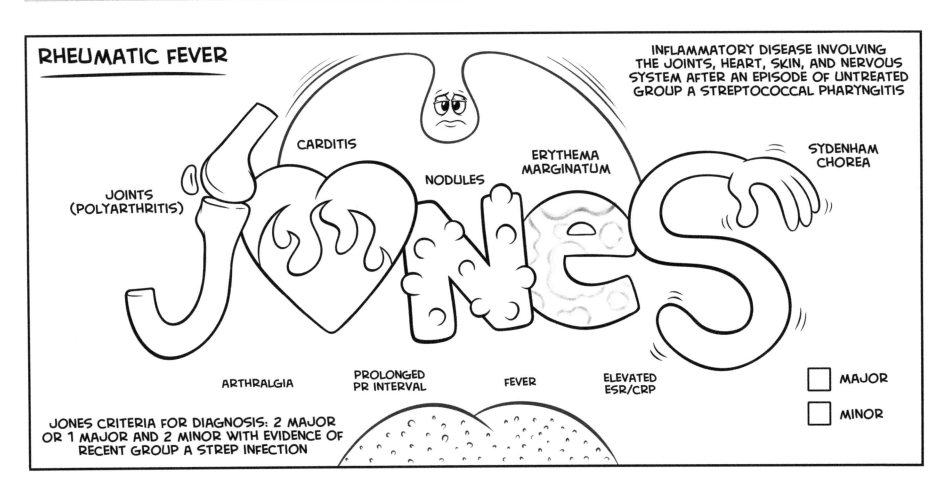

RHEUMATIC FEVER

INFLAMMATORY DISEASE INVOLVING THE JOINTS, HEART, SKIN, AND NERVOUS SYSTEM AFTER AN EPISODE OF UNTREATED GROUP A STREPTOCOCCAL PHARYNGITIS

JOINTS (POLYARTHRITIS)

CARDITIS

NODULES

ERYTHEMA MARGINATUM

SYDENHAM CHOREA

ARTHRALGIA

PROLONGED PR INTERVAL

FEVER

ELEVATED ESR/CRP

MAJOR

MINOR

JONES CRITERIA FOR DIAGNOSIS: 2 MAJOR OR 1 MAJOR AND 2 MINOR WITH EVIDENCE OF RECENT GROUP A STREP INFECTION

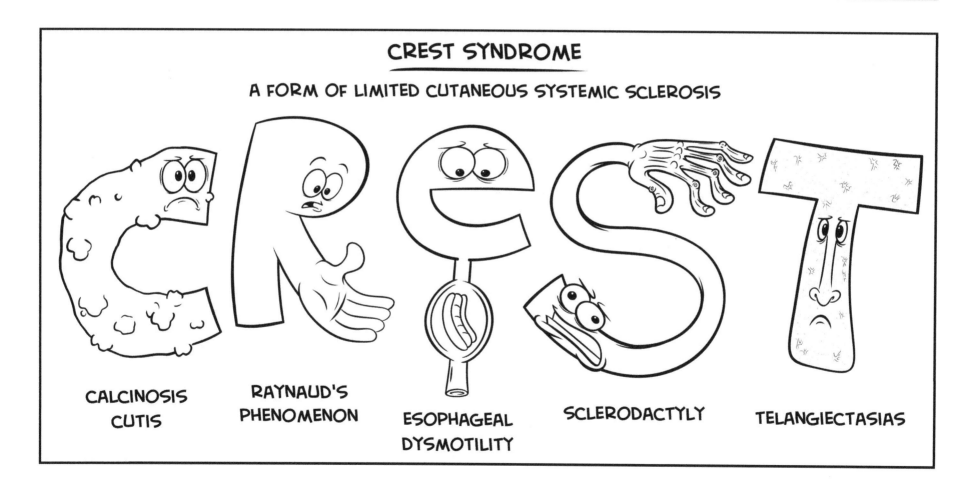

CREST SYNDROME

A FORM OF LIMITED CUTANEOUS SYSTEMIC SCLEROSIS

CALCINOSIS CUTIS

RAYNAUD'S PHENOMENON

ESOPHAGEAL DYSMOTILITY

SCLERODACTYLY

TELANGIECTASIAS

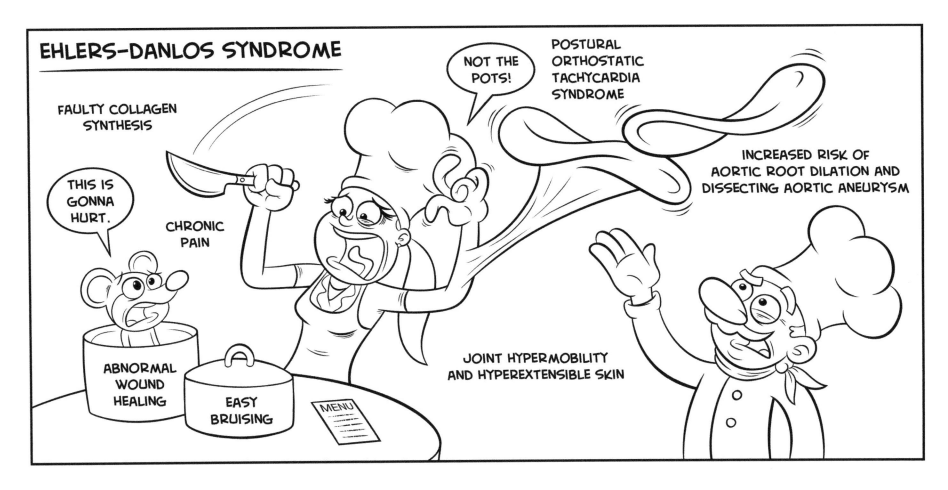

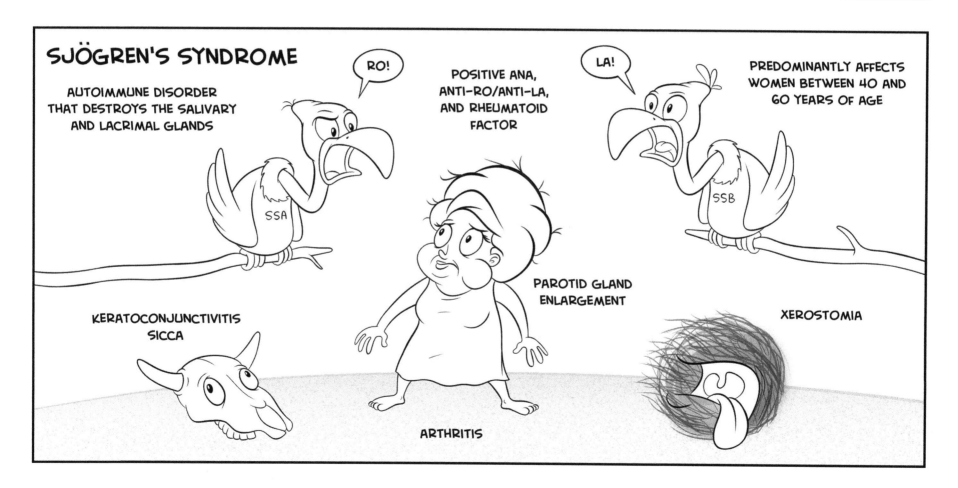

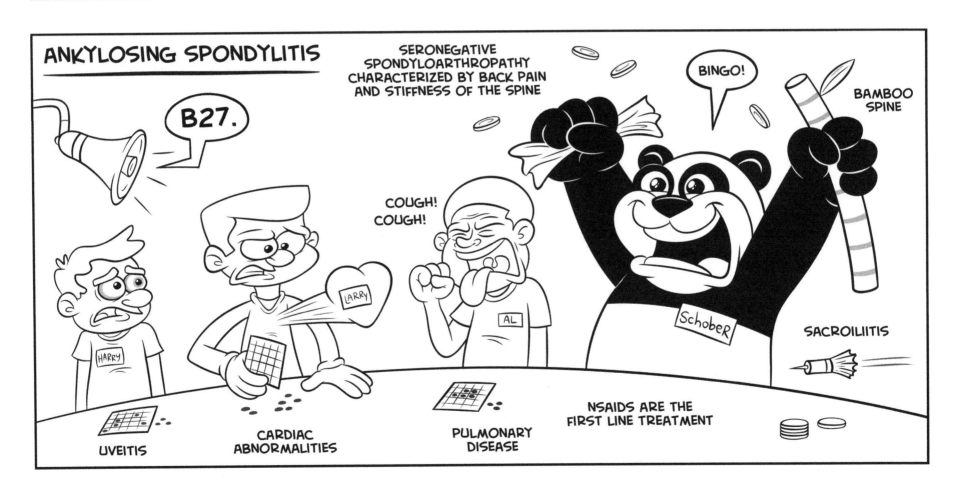

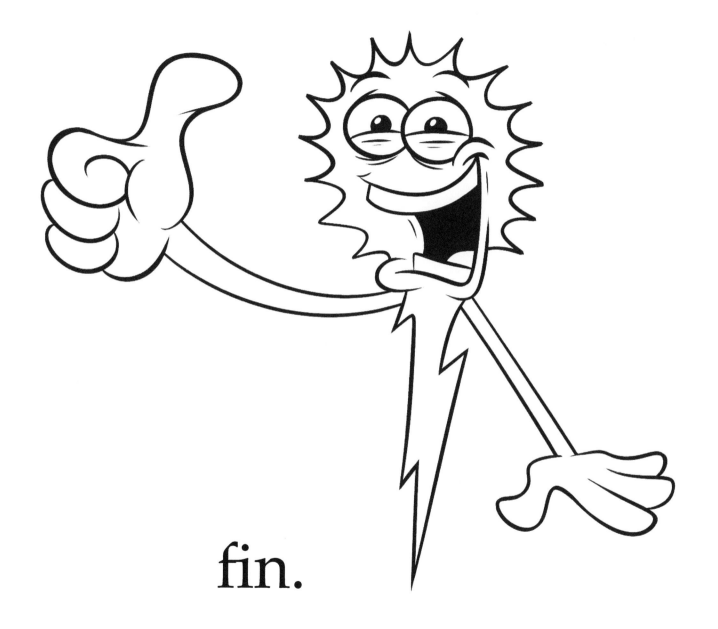

fin.

ABOUT THE AUTHOR

Jorge Muniz is the author and illustrator of *Medcomic: The Most Entertaining Way to Study Medicine* and *Sparkson's Illustrated Guide to ECG Interpretation*. He is a board certified PA from Orlando, Florida. He earned his Bachelor's degree in Biology in 2009 at George Mason University in Fairfax, Virginia. In 2013, he went on to complete his Master's degree in Medical Sciences at Nova Southeastern University (NSU) in Orlando, Florida.

Upon graduation from NSU, Jorge worked in the hospital setting in the field of orthopedic surgery. In 2015, he switched specialties to internal medicine, focusing on outpatient care. In 2018, Jorge embarked on a new journey to return to the hospital and become a cardiac electrophysiology PA.

Jorge has passions for art, education, entertainment, and medicine. His illustrations are influenced by old cartoons from his childhood. He is grateful for the opportunity to share these passions in a unique way and make a positive impact in communities around the world.

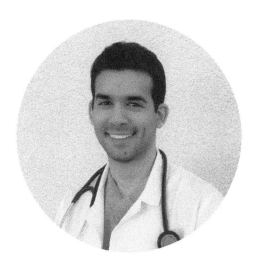

INDEX

CPSIA information can be obtained
at www.ICGtesting.com
Printed in the USA
BVHW021645101218
535253BV00005B/35/P